Trainee Workbook for Mental Health Approaches to Intellectual/Developmental Disability

Robert J. Fletcher, DSW, ACSW, NADD-CC
Daniel Baker, PhD, NADD-CC
Juanita St Croix, BSc
Melissa Cheplic, MPH

Copyright © 2015 NADD Press

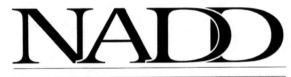 An association for persons with developmental disabilities and mental health needs.

132 Fair Street
Kingston, New York 12401

All rights reserved.

No part of this book may be reproduced, stored in a retrieval system or transmitted in any form by means of electronic, mechanical, photocopy, recording or otherwise, without written permission of NADD, 132 Fair Street, Kingston, New York 12401.

ISBN: 1-57256-141-6

Printed in the United States of America

Introduction to Trainee Workbook

Welcome to *Trainee Workbook for Mental Health Approaches to Intellectual/Developmental Disability*. This workbook is a companion to *Mental Health Approaches to Intellectual/Developmental Disability: A Resource for Trainers* and is designed to be given to all participants in workshops using the *Resource for Trainers*. The *Trainee Workbook* contains copies of all slides that will be used in your training, but does not include text explaining the slides. That information will be provided by your trainer. The *Trainee Workbook* does include space for you to record your own notes about the material. Each training module includes a pre-test to be taken prior to the training and a post-test to be taken after the training.

The *Resource for Trainers* and the *Trainee Workbook* provide training concerning the field of support for persons with intellectual or developmental disabilities (IDD) and mental health concerns. The material is arranged in ten modules. It is unlikely that a single training session would attempt to cover all modules.

Module I: What Is a Dual Diagnosis?

Module II: Building on the Basics: Understanding Assessment Practices in Dual Diagnosis

Module III: Mental Health Evaluations

Module IV: Signs and Symptoms of Mental Illness

Module V: From DM-ID to DM-ID-2

Module VI: Support Strategies

Module VII: Adapting Therapy for People with IDD

Module VIII: Childhood and Adolescence

Module IX: Aging

Module X: Inter-Systems Collaboration

As mentioned, the *Trainee Workbook* is a companion to the *Resource for Trainers*. The *Resource for Trainers* includes copies of the slides, extensive information about the content in the slides, and references for further study. In addition to preparing a trainer to offer workshops on topics concerning mental health and intellectual/developmental disability, *the Resource for Trainers* can be used for individual study or as a reference guide.

Module I

What Is a Dual Diagnosis?

Pre-Test

Module I: What Is a Dual Diagnosis

___ 1. Which of the following diagnostic criteria must NOT be met for a person to be considered to have an Intellectual or Developmental Disability?
   (a) Deficits in Intellectual Functioning
   (b) Inability to work productively at typical speeds
   (c) Deficits in Adaptive Functioning
   (d) Onset of deficits during the developmental period

___ 2. Which of these domains is NOT considered relevant to the diagnosis of an Intellectual or Developmental Disability?
   (a) Vocal domain
   (b) Conceptual domain
   (c) Social domain
   (d) Practical domain

___ 3. Which of these is a common type of Intellectual or Developmental Disability?
   (a) Lovecraft Syndrome
   (b) Zander Disorder
   (c) Aminesis
   (d) Fragile X

___ 4. People with Autism Spectrum Disorder often have difficulties with which of the following?
   (a) Dependence on routine
   (b) Uneven development profiles
   (c) Behavior problems
   (d) All of the above

___ 5. What is a Behavioral Phenotype?
   (a) A type of disability
   (b) A type of mental illness
   (c) A characteristic repertoire associated with a genetic disorder
   (d) A diagnostic code

___ 6. Which of the following does not change when people occasionally experience mental health problems:
   (a) The level of intellectual functioning
   (b) The way they think and understand the world
   (c) The way they interrelate with other
   (d) The emotions and feelings they experience

7. People with Intellectual or Developmental Disability and Mental Illness:
   (a) Almost never work

Slide 1

**Mental Health Approaches to
Intellectual/Developmental Disability:
A Resource for Trainers**

Dr. Robert J. Fletcher
    Founder and CEO, NADD

Dr. Dan Baker
    The Boggs Center, Rutgers RWJMS

Juanita St. Croix,
    Regional Support Associates/The
    Southern Network of Specialized Care

Melissa Cheplic, MPH
    The Boggs Center, Rutgers RWJMS

Slide 2

Module I

What is a Dual Diagnosis?

Slide 3

CONCEPT OF DUAL DIAGNOSIS

Slide 4

This module covers basic information about the nature of Mental Health disorders among persons with Intellectual or Developmental Disabilities (IDD). The following content will be covered: definitions of IDD and mental illness, prevalence, indicators, common syndromes, characteristics, vulnerability factors, similarities and differences between MI and IDD.

Slide 5

Learning Objectives

- Define IDD
- Articulate prevalence rates
- Identify and describe 3 of the common syndromes
- Identify the four levels of severity
- Describe what is meant by "behavioral phenotype"
- Define MI
- Articulate prevalence rates
- Identify and describe DSM usage
- Define Dual Diagnosis
- Articulate prevalence rates
- Describe characteristics
- Describe vulnerability risk factors
- Articulate the similarities and differences between MI and IDD
- Describe four characteristics of persons with IDD/MI
- Describe vulnerability risk factors

Slide 6

Concept Of Dual Diagnosis

- Co-Existence of Two Disabilities:
  Intellectual/Developmental Disability (IDD) and Mental Illness (MI)

- Both IDD and Mental Health disorders should be assessed and diagnosed

- All needed treatments and supports should be available, effective and accessible

Slide 7

Terminology

The DSM 5 was published in May 2013 with many changes in diagnostic criteria and terminology.

One of these is the change from the term "mental retardation" from DSM –IV to the term "intellectual disability" or "intellectual developmental disorder." This change better reflects terminology changes by medical, educational, service professionals and advocacy groups.

Slide 8

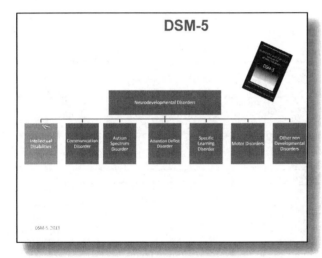

DSM-5

Neurodevelopmental Disorders: Intellectual Disabilities, Communication Disorder, Autism Spectrum Disorder, Attention Deficit Disorder, Specific Learning Disorder, Motor Disorders, Other non Developmental Disorders

Slide 9

Intellectual Developmental Disability – Diagnostic Criteria

Intellectual/Developmental Disability

Following 3 diagnostic criteria must be met:

A. Deficits in intellectual functioning such as reasoning, problem solving, planning. Abstract thinking, academic learning and learning from experience, confirmed by both clinical assessment and individualized standardized testing;

B. Deficits in adaptive functioning that result in failure to meet developmental and sociocultural standards for personal independence and social responsibility. Without ongoing support, the adaptive deficits limit functioning in one or more activities of daily life, such as communication, social participation and independent living, across multiple environments such as home, school, work, and community.

C. Onset of intellectual and adaptive deficits during the developmental period.

Slide 10

Intellectual Developmental Disability – Three Domains

Disorder Characteristics: Three Domains

Intellectual/Developmental Disability involves impairments of general mental abilities that impact adaptive functioning in three domains, or areas. These domains determine how well an individual copes with everyday tasks:

- The Conceptual Domain includes skills in language, reading, writing, math, reasoning, knowledge and memory.
- The Social Domain refers to empathy, social judgment, interpersonal communication skills, the ability to make and maintain friendships, and similar capacities
- The Practical Domain centers on self-management in areas such as personal care, job responsibilities, money management, recreation, and organizing school and work tasks.

Slide 11

Deficits in Adaptive Functioning

- **Self-care**
- Language and communication
- **Community use**
- Independent living skills

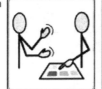

Slide 12

Deficits in Adaptive Functioning
(continued)

- **Socialization skills**
- Health and safety
- **Work**
- Self-direction

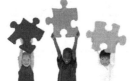

Slide 13

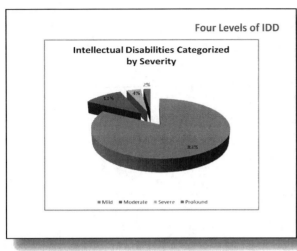

Four Levels of IDD

Intellectual Disabilities Categorized by Severity

■ Mild ■ Moderate ■ Severe ■ Profound

Slide 14

Four Levels of IDD

Mild: 80 – 85% of people with IDD
- Slower than normal development in all areas
- Unusual physiology rare
- Typical skill repertoire includes
  - practical skills
  - literacy skills
  - tasks of daily living/self-care
  - social skills

Slide 15

Four Levels of IDD

Moderate: 10 – 12 % of people with IDD

- Noticeable delays, particularly speech
- May have unusual physiology
- Typical skills repertoire includes
  - simple communication skills
  - simple health and safety skills
  - some tasks of daily living/self-care
  - independence in the community in familiar places

Slide 16

Four Levels of IDD

Severe: 3-4% of people with IDD

- Significant delays in some areas
- May walk late
- Limited expressive communication skills
- Typical skills repertoire includes
    - daily routines and repetitive activities
    - less complex tasks of daily living/self-care
    - social skills with support and supervision

DSM-5, 2013

Slide 17

Four Levels of IDD

Profound: 1-2% of people with IDD

- Significant delays in all areas
- Congenital abnormalities present
- Need close supervision
- Require specialized/attendant care
- May respond to regular physical and social activity
- Need intensive support to do self-care and activities of daily living

DSM-5, 2013

Slide 18

Exercise and Discussion

- What do you know about each of the severity levels of IDD (mild, moderate, severe, profound)?

- What is your personal experience with someone who has a disability?

Slide 19

Intellectual/Developmental Disability - Causes

Thousands of Causes

- Chromosomal abnormalities
- Environmental genetic abnormalities
- Infections
- Metabolic issues/disorders
- Nutritional deficiencies/abnormalities
- Toxicity
- Trauma (Prenatal and perinatal)
- Unknown

Slide 20

Common Types of Intellectual Developmental Disability

- **Down syndrome**
- Fragile X
- **Autism Spectrum Disorders (ASD)**
- Fetal Alcohol Spectrum Disorder (FASD)

Slide 21

Down Syndrome

Down syndrome is a genetic condition causing a set of delays in physical and intellectual development as a result of having an extra copy of chromosome 21.

MODULE I

Slide 22

Down Syndrome

All people with Down syndrome experience cognitive delays, but the effect is usually mild to moderate.

NDSS, 2012

Slide 23

Down Syndrome

People who have Down syndrome have increased risk for certain medical conditions such as:

- congenital heart defects
- respiratory and hearing problems
- Alzheimer's disease
- childhood leukemia
- thyroid conditions

A few of the common physical traits of Down syndrome are low muscle tone, small stature, an upward slant to the eyes, and a single deep crease across the center of the palm.

NDSS, 2012

Slide 24

Fragile X

- Fragile X syndrome is a genetic condition that causes a range of developmental problems including learning disabilities and cognitive impairment.
- Usually, males are more severely affected by this disorder than females.
- Fragile X syndrome does not always cause intellectual disability, but most people who have Fragile X have a mild or moderate intellectual disability.

OM-ID, 2007

Slide 25

Autism Spectrum Disorder

Autism Spectrum Disorder (ASD) is a complex condition that impacts normal brain development and affects a person's social relationships, communication, interests and behavior across multiple contexts. ASD is a single condition with different levels of symptom severity.

Slide 26

Autism Spectrum Disorder

Parts of the Brain Affected by Autism

Cerebral Cortex:
A thin layer of gray matter on the surface of the cerebral hemispheres. Two thirds of this area is deep in the tissues and folds. This area of the brain is responsible for higher mental functions, general movement, perception and behavioral reactions.

Amygdala:
This is responsible for all emotional responses including aggressive behavior.

Basal Ganglia:
This is gray masses deep within the cerebral hemisphere that connects the cerebrum and the cerebellum. It helps regulate automatic movement.

Hippocampus:
This makes it possible to remember new information and recent events.

Corpus Callosum:
This consists of closely packed bundles of fibers that connect the right and left hemispheres of the brain and allows them to communicate with one another.

Brain Stem:
The Brain Stem is located in front of the cerebellum and serves as a relay station, passing messages between various parts of the body and the cerebral cortex. It controls the primitive functions of the body essential to survival including breathing and heart rate.

Cerebellum:
This is located at the back of the brain. It fine tunes motor activity, regulates balance, body movements, coordination and the muscles used for speaking.

Slide 27

Autism Spectrum Disorder

ASD is characterized by:

- Persistent deficits in social communication and social interaction across multiple contexts

And

- Restricted, repetitive patterns of behavior, interests, or activities

Slide 28

Autism Spectrum Disorder

People who have an autism spectrum disorder often have difficulties with:

- Social relationships
- Transitions
- Communication / language
- Perseveration on interests and activities
- Dependence on routine
- Abnormal responses to sensory stimulation
- Behavior problems
- Variability of intellectual functioning
- Uneven development profile
- Difficulties in sleeping, toileting and eating
- Immune irregularities
- Nutritional deficiencies
- Gastrointestinal problems

Slide 29

Autism Spectrum Disorder

ASD is typically noticed in the first or second year of life with:

- delay or abnormality in language and play,
- repetitive behaviors, such as spinning things or lining up small objects,
- or unusual interests such as preoccupations with stop signs or ceiling fans.

Slide 30

Autism Spectrum Disorder

Common Strengths

- Non-verbal reasoning skills
- Reading skills
- Perceptual motor skills
- Drawing skills
- Computer interest and skills
- Exceptional memory
- Visual spatial abilities
- Music skills

Slide 31

Autism Spectrum Disorder

Deficits in social communication can be observed in these areas:
- Delay in development of spoken language (no speech)
- Lack of responses to the communications of others
- Pronoun confusion (e.g., I vs. You)
- Stereotypical and repetitive use of language (e.g., using lines from a favorite movie to communicate)
- Idiosyncratic use of words and phrases (e.g., always salutes and says "Yes sir" when given a direction)
- Abnormalities in pitch, stress, rate, rhythm, and intonation of speech

McEvoy, Rogers, and Pennington, 2006

Slide 32

Autism Spectrum Disorder

Deficits in social interaction can be observed in these areas:
- Failure to initiate or sustain conversations (e.g., turn taking)
- Serious deficits in the ability to make friendships
- Failure to respond to their names when called
- Appearing not to listen when spoken to
- Difficulty identifying boundaries of others

McEvoy, Rogers, and Pennington, 2006

Slide 33

Autism Spectrum Disorder

Restricted repetitive behaviors, interests and activities may be observed as:
- Perseveration of interests and activities – people who have ASD typically have a narrow range of interests
- Repetitive, stereotyped body movements such as hand flicking, spinning or rocking
- Perseverations might extend to food
- Dependence on routine

McEvoy, Rogers, and Pennington, 2006

Slide 34

Fetal Alcohol Spectrum Disorder (FASD)

FASD is a term used to describe a range of disabilities caused by pre-natal exposure to alcohol.

Astley & Clarren, 2002

Slide 35

FASD

The 4-digit Diagnostic Code provides a reproducible, objective, consistent and precise method for the diagnosis of FAS. Four criteria are assessed, quantified and assigned a rating of 1 to 4 for each criteria, depending on the degree of abnormality:

- impaired growth;
- facial abnormalities;
- abnormal brain function; and
- degree of maternal drinking.

Astley & Clarren, 1999

Slide 36

FASD

While each person impacted by FASD is unique, brain damage typically results in various dysfunctional behavioral symptoms commonly found with this disability.

Astley & Clarren, 2002

Slide 37

Preventable *Secondary* Characteristics — FASD

In the absence of accurate diagnosis, patterns of defensive behaviors commonly develop over time. These are called secondary characteristics of FASD.
- Fatigue, tantrums
- Irritability, frustration, anger, aggression
- Fear, anxiety, avoidance, withdrawal
- Shut down, lying, running away
- Trouble at home, school, and community
- Legal trouble
- Drug / Alcohol abuse
- Mental health problems (depression, self injury, suicidal tendencies)

Streissguth et al., 2004

Slide 38

Genetics & IDD

- 283 Causes of IDD identified in 1994
- 1200 + Genetic Causes of IDD in 2013
- Prenatal causes dominated diagnosis

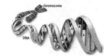

Slide 39

Phenotype and Genotypes

<u>Definition of Phenotype:</u>

The phenotype of a genetic syndrome is the set of physical characteristics produced by a genetic abnormality or genotype (DM-ID, 2009).

<u>Definition of Behavioral Phenotype:</u>

The specific and characteristic repertoire exhibited by people with a genetic disorder (Flint & Yule, 1994).

Slide 40

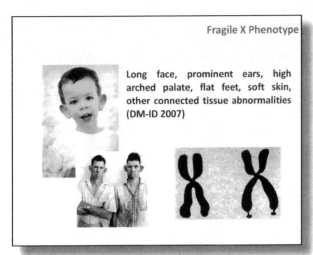

Fragile X Phenotype

Long face, prominent ears, high arched palate, flat feet, soft skin, other connected tissue abnormalities (DM-ID 2007)

Slide 41

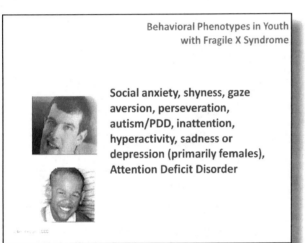

Behavioral Phenotypes in Youth with Fragile X Syndrome

Social anxiety, shyness, gaze aversion, perseveration, autism/PDD, inattention, hyperactivity, sadness or depression (primarily females), Attention Deficit Disorder

Slide 42

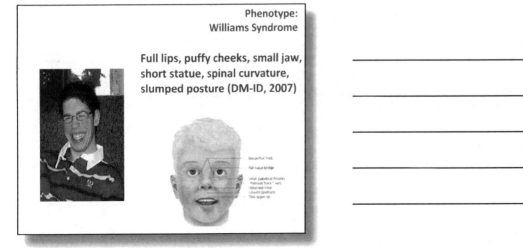

Phenotype: Williams Syndrome

Full lips, puffy cheeks, small jaw, short statue, spinal curvature, slumped posture (DM-ID, 2007)

Slide 43

Behavioral Phenotypes in Youth with Williams Syndrome

Anxiety, fears, phobias, inattention, hyperactivity, social disinhibiting, overly friendly, indiscriminate relating, Attention Deficit Disorder

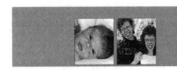

Slide 44

Prader-Willi Phenotype

Hyperphagia, obesity, small hands and feet, dysmorphic facial features (DM-ID, 2007)

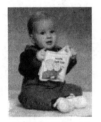
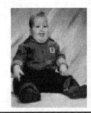

Slide 45

with Prader-Willi

- Hyperphagia, non-food obsessions & compulsions, skin-picking, temper tantrums, perseveration, stubbornness, under activity, OCD, Affective Disorders

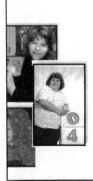

Slide 46

Down Syndrome Phenotype

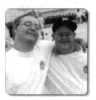

Small head, upward slant eyes, broad neck, hearing loss, obesity, gastrointestinal problems (DM-ID, 2007)

Slide 47

Behavioral Phenotypes in Youth with Down Syndrome

Noncompliance, stubbornness, inattention, over activity, argumentative, withdrawn (depression and dementia among adults), ADHD

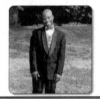

Slide 48

Behavioral Phenotypes

Behavioral phenotypes
- Are not set in stone
- Look at syndromes rather than set diagnoses
- Behavioral manifestations arise from the interaction of genes and environment
- Present a wide range of symptoms
- Used as clues not as expectations

Slide 49

Mental Health Problems vs. Mental Illness

People occasionally experience mental health problems that may:

- Change the way they think and understand the world around them
- Change the way they interrelate with others
- Change the emotions and feelings they have

These changes can have a short-term impact on the way they deal with day-to-day life.

However, if the impact is very great (ongoing problems with repeated relapse episodes) then we consider the possibility of mental illness.

Slide 50

What Is Mental Illness (MI)?

- MI is a psychiatric condition that disrupts a person's thinking, feeling, mood, ability to relate to others, and can impair daily functioning.

- MI can affect persons of any age, race, religion, income, or level of intelligence.

- The DSM 5 or the DM-ID provide diagnostic criteria for mental disorders.

DSM 5, 2013

Slide 51

What Is Mental Illness? (cont.)

Mental illness is a biological process that affects the brain. Some refer to it as a brain disorder.

DSM 5, 2013

Slide 52

Vulnerabilities

Mental illnesses (mental disorders) can also be defined as a variety of psychiatric conditions which may be a result of vulnerabilities in:

- Environment
- Biology
- Psychosocial factors

Slide 53

Definition Of Mental Illness In Persons With Intellectual/Developmental Disability

Criteria

1. When behavior is abnormal by virtue of quantitative or qualitative differences.

2. When behavior cannot be explained on the basis of developmental delay alone.

3. When behavior causes significant impairment in functioning.

Slide 54

A Summary Of Similarities And Differences Between Intellectual/Developmental Disability (IDD) & Mental Illness (MI)

IDD: refers to sub-average functional intellect
MI: has nothing to do with intellect

IDD: incidence: 1-2% of general population
MI: incidence: 16-20% of general population

IDD: present at birth or occurs before age 18
MI: may have its onset at any age (usually late adolescent)

Slide 55

A Summary Of Similarities And Differences Between Intellectual/Developmental Disability (IDD) & Mental Illness (MI)

IDD: functional intellectual impairment is permanent
MI: often temporary and may be reversible and is often cyclic

IDD: a person can usually be expected to behave rationally at his or her developmental level
MI: a person may vacillate between normal and irrational behavior, displaying degrees of each

Slide 56

Exercise

What did you learn from this section regarding people who have IDD/MI?

Slide 57

Comparison Between IDD and MI

Intellectual/Developmental Disability	Mental Illness
Below-average ability to learn and to use information	Inappropriate thought processes &/or emotions
Before adulthood	Can occur anytime in a person's life
Refers to sub-average functional intellect	Has nothing to do with intellect
Lifelong. There is no cure.	May be temporary, cyclic, or episodic. May be curable
Services involve training and education not medication	Services involve therapy and medication
Is not psychiatric in nature	Diagnosed illnesses such as Depression, Schizophrenia, Bi-Polar Disorder
Impairments in social skills and adaptations	Does not necessarily impact social competence
Behavior is usually rational	Behavior may vacillate between normal and irrational

Slide 58

Prevalence of MI in IDD

Two to four times
a typical population
(Corbett 1979)

40% of people with IDD have co-occurring MI
(Einfeld and Tongue, 1996)

44% of people with IDD have MI
(Nci, 20145)

Slide 59

Prevalence in US

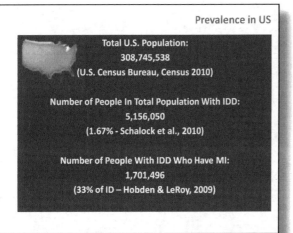

Total U.S. Population:
308,745,538
(U.S. Census Bureau, Census 2010)

Number of People In Total Population With IDD:
5,156,050
(1.67% - Schalock et al., 2010)

Number of People With IDD Who Have MI:
1,701,496
(33% of ID – Hobden & LeRoy, 2009)

Slide 60

Prevalence Canada

Total Canada Population
35,141,542
(Government of Canada, Statistics Canada, 2015)

Number of People in Total Population with IDD:
586,864
(1.67% - Schalock et al., 2010)

Number of People With IDD Who Have MI:
193,665
(33% of ID – Hobden & LeRoy, 2009)

Slide 61

Signs a person with IDD may have an MI — Indicators

• Increased anxiety, panic or fright	• Excessive reactivity / moodiness
• Hearing, seeing, feeling imaginary things (hearing voices is not the same as talking to oneself for company, to process thoughts, or self-talk to reduce anxiety)	• Memory problems (worsening memory or change in memory)
• Need for instant fulfillment / gratification	• Accelerated speech patterns
• Unusual sleep patterns (insomnia or lengthy periods of sleep)	• Changes in appetite (loss of weight or increase in weight)
• False beliefs (delusional thinking or paranoia)	• Heightened emotional sensitivity

Slide 62

Signs a person with IDD may have an MI Continued

• Decline in personal hygiene	• Self-isolation
• Inappropriate expressive reactions	• Lingering sadness
• Family history of mental illness	• Self-injurious behavior
• A functional or behavioral change	• Suicidal ideation

Slide 63

Consider this person

Nguyen is a 48 year old man with Down syndrome. He recently has begun to refuse previously enjoyed activities and occasionally becomes agitated when prompted to get ready for work in the morning, preferring to stay in bed all day with the lights out. His family and in home staff are frustrated with him and one person has stated that he is just plain lazy. Could this be depression?

Slide 64

Characteristics of People with IDD/MI

High Vulnerability to Stress

The impact of a minimally or moderately stressful situation can be experienced as significant.

Slide 65

Characteristics Of People With IDD/MI

- Challenges with coping skills
- Stress management difficulties
- Fewer wellness opportunities
- Frequently lack the basic skills required for everyday living; e.g., budgeting money, using public transportation, doing laundry, preparing meals, etc.

Slide 66

Characteristics Of People With IDD/MI

Extreme Dependency

Often experience themselves as quite helpless, thus requiring massive support from families or care providers to live successfully

Slide 67

Characteristics of People with IDD/MI

Difficulty with Interpersonal Relationships

- With some exceptions, people with IDD/MI often have great difficulty in developing and maintaining close relationships with others.
- These interpersonal relationship problems can result in disruption in school, home, work, and social environments.

Slide 68

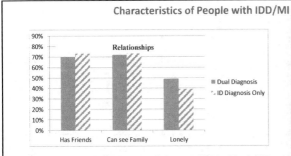

Characteristics of People with IDD/MI — Relationships

People with dual diagnosis were less likely to report having friends (70% vs. 75%) and being able to see family whenever desired (72% vs. 83%) than were those with IDD only. On the other hand, they were considerably more likely to report feeling lonely (49%) than were people with diagnosis of only IDD (39%).

Slide 69

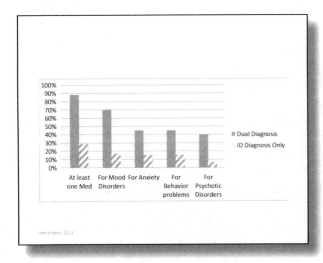

Slide 70

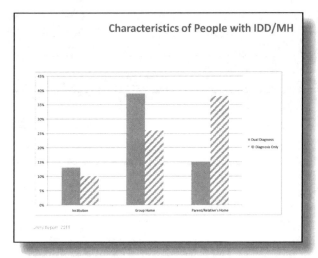

Slide 71

Characteristics of People with IDD/MI

Difficulty Working in the Competitive Job Market

People with IDD/MI often have difficulty working in a competitive employment. They may have frequent job changes interspersed with long periods of unemployment.

Slide 72

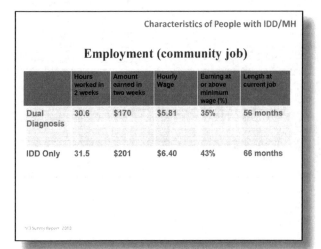

Slide 73

Characteristics of People with IDD/MI

- People with IDD/MI may learn more slowly.
- They may have difficulty recalling information – especially newly required information.

Slide 74

Characteristics of People with IDD/MI

- May have difficulty focusing, may have shortened attention span
- Difficulty in understanding some abstract concepts
- May have difficulty in considering alternative solutions. For example, may see things in "black and white" terms.

Slide 75

Characteristics of People with IDD/MI

- May have difficulty generalizing skills sets
- Developed skill sets may be very task specific
- Passive learning style which may make it difficult for the trainer to know what information is being retained
- Low expectations due to past difficulties. "Self fulfilled prophecy"- the individual believes he/she can not learn, thus preventing learning.

Slide 76

Characteristics of People with IDD/MI

Exercise

Can you share examples of what might assist a person with IDD through some of the learning issues on the previous slide?

Slide 77

Characteristics of People with IDD/MI

- May "perseverate" on some things
- Much harder to focus on things that are too difficult
- Problems with cognitive rigidity:
  ❖ Difficulty changing from one task to another
  ❖ Difficulty accepting alternative solutions or explanations
  ❖ Difficulty shifting focus of attention

Slide 78

Characteristics of People with IDD/MI

- Being different from peers
- Losses rather than gains
- Social isolation although mainstreamed
- Rejected by peers
- Failure experiences dominate school histories
- Low social status

Slide 79

Characteristics of People with IDD/MI

- Outer directed personality orientation
  - look to others rather than selves for problem solution
- Aberrant social styles:
  ❖ Too wary or too disinhibited
  ❖ Low expectancy or enjoyment of success

Slide 80

Characteristics Of People With IDD/MI

- Low self-esteem
- Distrust of self
- Sadness, depression, dependency & withdrawal
- Helplessness
- Impulsivity

Slide 81

Vulnerability Factors for Developing Psychiatric Disorders in People with IDD

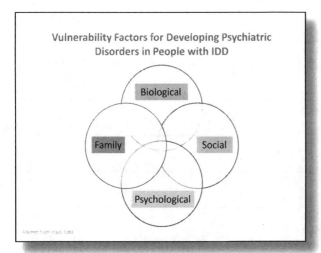

Slide 82

Vulnerability Factors

People with IDD are at increased risk of developing psychiatric disorders due to complex interaction of multiple factors:

- Biological
- Psychological
- Social
- Family

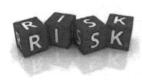

Slide 83

Vulnerability Factors

Vulnerability factors for psychiatric disorders:

Biological

- Brain damage/epilepsy
- Vision/hearing impairments
- Physical illnesses/disabilities
- Genetic/familial conditions
- Drugs/alcohol abuse
- Medication/physical treatments

Slide 84

Vulnerability Factors

Vulnerability factors for psychiatric disorders:

Psychological

- Rejection/deprivation/abuse
- Life events/separations/losses
- Poor problem-solving/coping strategies
- Social/emotional/sexual vulnerabilities
- Poor self-acceptance/low self-esteem
- Devaluation/disempowerment

Slide 85

Vulnerability Factors

Vulnerability factors for psychiatric disorders:

Social

- Negative attitudes/expectations
- **Stigmatization/prejudice/social exclusion**
- Poor supports/relationships/networks
- **Inappropriate environments/services**
- Financial/legal disadvantages

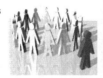

Slide 86

Vulnerability Factors

Vulnerability factors for psychiatric disorders:

Family

- Diagnostic/bereavement issues
- **Life-cycle transitions/crises**
- Stress/adaptation to disability
- **Limited social/community networks**
- Difficulties "letting go"

Slide 87

Exercise

How can we support someone in improving their quality of life when one or more of these risk factors are present?

MODULE I

Post-Test

Module I: What Is a Dual Diagnosis

___ 1. Which of the following diagnostic criteria must NOT be met for a person to be considered to have an Intellectual or Developmental Disability?
   (a) Deficits in Intellectual Functioning
   (b) Inability to work productively at typical speeds
   (c) Deficits in Adaptive Functioning
   (d) Onset of deficits during the developmental period

___ 2. Which of these domains is NOT considered relevant to the diagnosis of an Intellectual or Developmental Disability?
   (a) Vocal domain
   (b) Conceptual domain
   (c) Social domain
   (d) Practical domain

___ 3. Which of these is a common type of Intellectual or Developmental Disability?
   (a) Lovecraft Syndrome
   (b) Zander Disorder
   (c) Aminesis
   (d) Fragile X

___ 4. People with Autism Spectrum Disorder often have difficulties with which of the following?
   (a) Dependence on routine
   (b) Uneven development profiles
   (c) Behavior problems
   (d) All of the above

___ 5. What is a Behavioral Phenotype?
   (a) A type of disability
   (b) A type of mental illness
   (c) A characteristic repertoire associated with a genetic disorder
   (d) A diagnostic code

___ 6. Which of the following does not change when people occasionally experience mental health problems:
   (a) The level of intellectual functioning
   (b) The way they think and understand the world
   (c) The way they interrelate with other
   (d) The emotions and feelings they experience

___ 7. People with Intellectual or Developmental Disability and Mental Illness:
   (a) Almost never work
   (b) Can only work in a sheltered environment
   (c) Have more difficulty working than the average person with IDD
   (d) Experience very few difficulties in employment

___ 8. Which of the following is NOT a vulnerability for developing psychiatric disorders in persons with IDD?
   (a) Social
   (b) Family
   (c) Psychological
   (d) Vaccinations

___ 9. What of the following is a reasonable percentage of people with Intellectual or Developmental Disability ikely to also have a mental health disorder?
   (a) 0%
   (b) 8%
   (c) 40%
   (d) 80%

___ 10. Which of the following is similar between IDD and MI?
   (a) Intellectual functioning
   (b) Time of onset
   (c) Difficulties in social adjustment
   (d) All of the above.

Module II

Building on the Basics: Understanding Assessment Practices in Dual Diagnosis

Pre-Test

Module II: Integrated Assessment

___ 1. Which of the following is NOT an example of a medical condition that contributes to problem or maladaptive behavior?
    (a) Diabetes
    (b) Urinary tract infection
    (c) Acid reflux
    (d) None of the above

___ 2. Fill in the blank: The _____ of assessment considers the dynamic influence of four traditional models to arrive at a multi-modal assessment of maladaptive behavior that considers multiple determinants and how each may contribute to the function of behavior.
    (a) Communication Model
    (b) Behavior Model
    (c) Integrative Model
    (d) Medical Model

___ 3. Possible functions of challenging behavior in people with IDD/MI can include:
    (a) To gain attention from others.
    (b) To escape or avoid demands.
    (c) To obtain tangible items or opportunities
    (d) All of the above

___ 4. Best practice in assessment and diagnosis for people with IDD/MI refers to
    (a) The Bio-psychosocial model
    (b) Behavior analysis
    (c) Mental health assessments
    (d) An annual physical completed by a regulated health professional

___ 5. The bio-psychosocial model:
    (a) Incorporates the effects of biomedical and psychological factors and how these influences interrelate.
    (b) Does not require the review of existing data or background information to contribute to the assessment process.
    (c) Recognizes that clinical interview can be completed by reviewing the documented history and reports compiled about the person.
    (d) Recognizes that mental health is defined only by the relative absence of psychological distress.

___ 6. Which of the premises about people with an IDD is false?
  (a) The full range of psychiatric conditions expressed in the general population is also represented in persons with IDD.
  (b) Persons with IDD are considered to have a lower prevalence rate of MI than the general population.
  (c) Persons with an IDD may tell a clinician or care provider what he or she thinks they want to hear or agree to things to avoid the risk of disapproval.
  (d) None of the above.

___ 7. One of the first steps to completing a functional assessment is
  (a) Assessing the effectiveness of different approaches on the target behavior
  (b) Describing the target behavior; assigning an operational definition.
  (c) Identifying the patterns of triggers to help figure out how a behavior is maintained.
  (d) Understanding the behavior from the perspective of the person who directly observes it and the problem it causes for other people.

___ 8. The Integrative Model posits that
  (a) Problem behaviors can be completely attributed to the existence of a co-existing medical problem.
  (b) There are often multiple determinants that influence the expression of maladaptive behavior.
  (c) Manipulating the environment in such a way as to increase or decrease problem behavior assists in identifying the needs/emotions or a person with IDD.
  (d) The most effective treatment of problem behavior is teaching communication skills.

___ 9. Which of the following is the most suggestive indicator that a behavior pattern may be the result of a mental illness?
  (a) The behavior never occurs when the person's favorite direct support professional is supporting him/her.
  (b) The person appears to be able to start and stop the behavior at will.
  (c) The behavior is exhibited only at home.
  (d) The behavior occurs in all environments; it is not just observed in specific settings.

___ 10. Which one of the following statements is accurate?
  (a) Medical problems in people with IDD are easily recognized.
  (b) Dental problems in people with IDD are easily recognized.
  (c) Rapid onset in a change in behavior patterns is likely because behavioral problems are directly associated with having the condition of IDD.
  (d) Causes of SIB in people with IDD can be related to an underlying medical condition.

Slide 1

> # Module II
>
> Building on the Basics:
> Understanding Assessment
> Practices in Dual Diagnosis

Slide 2

> CONCEPTUAL MODELS
> RELATED TO BEHAVIORAL
> PROBLEMS :
>
> AN INTEGRATED ASSESSMENT
> APPROACH

Slide 3

> This module includes content related to Conceptual Models Related to Behavior Problems: Integrative Approach, Functional Assessment of Behavior, and Assessment and Diagnostic Practices.

Slide 4

Learning Objectives

- Articulate the elements of behavioral, medical, communication, and physical model of problem behavior
- List possible functions of challenging behavior
- Describe what is meant by ABCs of behavior
- Understand the considerations of and steps for a functional assessment
- Describe the best practice in assessment and diagnosis
- List the components and importance of the Integrative Model
- Describe the diagnostic principles for completing a psychiatric diagnosis in a person with IDD
- Describe why medical causes of problem behavior are often under-diagnosed
- Summarize the importance of obtaining past and present medical history as it relates to problem behavior
- Describe three medical conditions that can present as psychiatric issues/behavioral problems
- Articulate the importance of medical assessments in the assessment process
- Provide three examples of medical conditions that contribute to maladaptive behavior.

Slide 5

An On-going Case Study

Cal is a Caucasian man in his late 20s (date of birth April 26, 1992) with diagnoses of moderate intellectual disability and Autism Spectrum Disorder. He has a history of seizures, but is not currently treated for his seizure disorder, and there are no seizures observed at the current time. Cal is a fun person; he is very physical and has a silly sense of humor. He has some spoken language, and also communicates through action. He likes staying active, and while he lives in a group home setting, he also has a very involved family. He attends a day program.

Slide 6

Conceptual Models Related to Behavioral Problems

Five Conceptual Models:

1. Medical Model
2. Communication Model
3. Behavioral Model
4. Psychiatric Model
5. Integrative Model (1-4)

Slide 7

Conceptual Models Related to Behavioral Problems

1. Medical Model

- Problem behaviors are exhibited because of co-existing medical problems
- Assessment of potential medical problems involves conducting a full medical work-up
- Treatment focuses on addressing the underlying medical problem

Engel, 1977

Slide 8

Conceptual Models Related to Behavioral Problems

2. Communication Model

- Views behavioral problems as reflecting "challenging behaviors" in persons who have deficits in language skills
- Treatment – teach communication skills
- Assessment focuses on evaluation of skills, deficits and communicative intent.

McClintock, Hall & Oliver, 2003

Slide 9

Conceptual Models Related to Behavioral Problems

3. Behavioral Model

- Problem behaviors are viewed according to learning principles
- Assessment identifies the antecedent and consequences of the problematic behavior
- Treatment focuses on changing or eliminating behavior though behavioral approaches
- Does not usually identify people's needs/emotions.

Baer, Wolf, & Risley, 1968

Slide 10

Conceptual Models Related to Behavioral Problems

4. Psychiatric Model

- Views problem behavior as a possible manifestation of a mental disorder
- Presentation of problem behaviors may be associated with a psychiatric disorder
- Assessment based on a bio-psycho-social model
- Treatment focuses on underlying psychiatric disorders

Slide 11

Conceptual Models Related to Behavioral Problems

5. Integrative Model

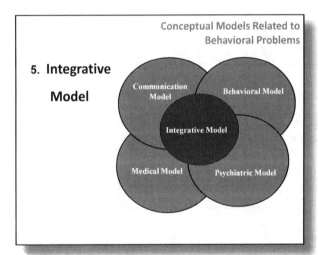

Slide 12

The Relationship of Challenging Behavior and IDD

Type of Model	Medical	Communication	Behavioral	Psychiatric
Assessment	Medical Evaluation by primary care physician	Standardized administered measure of expressive language	Functional Analysis	DM-ID
Problem Identification	Constipation	Speech and language impairment	Function/Need being met through behavior	Affective disorder, mania
Treatment	Medication for Bowel Movement (Laxative)	Functional communication skill training	Addressing unmet need, supporting appropriate behavior	Medication treatment, psychotherapy

Slide 13

Cal R.

Conceptual Models Related to Behavioral Problems

Cal does engage in some problem behaviors that can be severe at times, and has caused injury to staff persons. His team recommended that a Functional Assessment be completed to gain a better understanding of his support needs, as there is a clear need to change his behavior as it interferes with community access and is a risk to the health of others.

Slide 14

Functional Assessment of Problem Behavior

The Function of Behavior

Behaviors may persist because the individual...

- Enjoys the sensory experience – it feels better, satisfies a need or impulse (internal triggers, internal rewards)
- Escapes or avoids demands or things he or she doesn't like to do
- Gains attention from others
- Obtains tangible items or opportunities – access to something he or she prefers

Slide 15

Functional Assessment of Problem Behavior

Behavior Basics

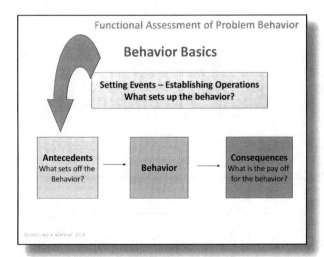

Setting Events – Establishing Operations
What sets up the behavior?

Antecedents (What sets off the Behavior?) → Behavior → Consequences (What is the pay off for the behavior?)

Slide 16

Functional Assessment of Problem Behavior

Considerations of Functional Assessment

- A pattern of behavior that repeats
- Understand why the behavior occurs
  - What are the Antecedents – Precursors, what "sets off" the behavior
  - Are there any Setting Events – things that set the person up to do the behavior
  - What are the Consequences – Outcomes, what does the person get as a result
- Is the behavior:
  - an attempt to communicate?
  - a way to avoid or obtain something?
  - the result of a medical condition or other factor?

Slide 17

Cal R.

One of the main concerns is that when he is in parking lots, he must search through the parking lot and find out if there are any convertibles. If he is blocked from completing the search, he will become very aggressive and essentially do whatever it takes to do a thorough search, even if it is a huge lot. His family reports that they simply avoided any large parking lot of any type while he lived at home. He does love convertibles, and has a collection of small convertible cars, and loves seeing them on tv. Numerous persons have referred to this as OCD, though he does not have a formal diagnosis of OCD. There is an ongoing debate, at time acrimonious, between care providers & family who consider this OCD and care providers & family who consider this a symptom of ASD.

Slide 18

Functional Assessment of Problem Behavior

The Steps to a Functional Assessment

- Describe what the target behavior is; the operational definition
- Interview the person or care providers
- Observe the person to see what else might be happening
- Use the interview and observation to make some guesses about the antecedents and consequences
- Identify antecedents, setting events, and consequences (outcomes)
- Look for patterns to identify function

Slide 19

Functional Assessment of Problem Behavior
Look for Patterns

- The same type of triggers tend to set the behavior off
- People respond in similar ways to maintain the behavior, the person gets the same kind of outcome
- Setting events (establishing operations) make behavior more likely to occur when trigger is present.
- The behavior doesn't have to happen every time the trigger is present but work enough to make the behavior "worth it" for the individual.

Slide 20

Functional Assessment of Problem Behavior
Go to the Experts
Involving direct caregivers in plan development

- Staff often work closest to and spend most time with people
- Encourage contributions, observations, hypotheses, ideas, intervention strategies
- Staff can identify trends and missing puzzle pieces that managers and behaviorists often cannot
- Foster control and confidence
- Promote participation and involvement in planning
- Consider opinions and answer questions
- Provide ongoing support and guidance

Slide 21

Cal R.

A Functional Assessment of Behavior was completed by a consultant that closely focused on the issues around parking lots and convertibles. It was determined that once Cal finds a convertible, he will continue on with the prior activities (i.e., he does not need to find a second convertible, though if it is a small parking lot he may briefly look for a second one). Additionally, if no convertible is found in the entire lot, he will continue with prior activities. This information was shared with his primary care physician at an appointment, which was also attended by team members and the consultant who completed the FA.

Slide 22

Cal R. - The outcome

The DM-ID (based on the DSM-IV-TR) was reviewed. At that point, the determination was made that there was no evidence of OCD, and that this pattern of behavior was a symptom of the ASD, and treatment was developed from a perspective informed by ASD, including the use of Social Stories and Structured Teaching.

Slide 23

Exercise

Review the case information on Slides 17 and 21 for Cal. List 2 ways staff involvement was instrumental in the process.

Slide 24

BEST PRACTICES

IN

ASSESSMENT AND DIAGNOSTIC

PROCEDURES

Slide 25

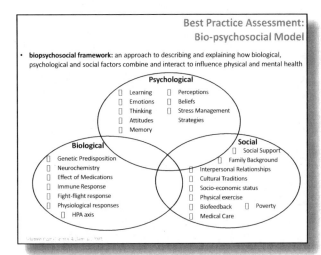

Best Practice Assessment: Bio-psychosocial Model

- **biopsychosocial framework:** an approach to describing and explaining how biological, psychological and social factors combine and interact to influence physical and mental health

Psychological
- Learning
- Emotions
- Thinking
- Attitudes
- Memory
- Perceptions
- Beliefs
- Stress Management Strategies

Biological
- Genetic Predisposition
- Neurochemistry
- Effect of Medications
- Immune Response
- Fight-flight response
- Physiological responses
- HPA axis

Social
- Social Support
- Family Background
- Interpersonal Relationships
- Cultural Traditions
- Socio-economic status
- Physical exercise
- Biofeedback
- Poverty
- Medical Care

Slide 26

Best Practice of Biopsychosocial Model

1. Incorporates the effects of biomedical and psychological factors and how these influences interrelate.

2. Uses assessment information to guide selection of diagnostically based interventions.

Slide 27

Best Practice of Bio-psycho-social Model

3. Identifies skills and related supports required by the individual to cope effectively with multiple biopsychosocial influences.

4. Proactive in focus.

5. Provides for translation of multiple modalities of influence in a common model.

Slide 28

Best Practice of Bio-psycho-social Model

6. Provides an integrated multimodal treatment plan.

7. Recognizes that mental health consists of both the presence of personal contentment, and the relative absence of psychological distress.

Slide 29

Best Practice Assessment: Bio-psycho-social Model

1. Review Reports

2. Interview Family

3. Interview Care Provider

4. Direct Observation

5. Clinical Interview

Slide 30

Mental Health Assessment & Managing the Interview

- Obtain records in advance
    - School, medical, development and family
- Become familiar with collateral informants who attend the interview
    - Parents, care provider, service coordinators
- Understand that the assessment interview can be stressful for all involved
    - Interviewer will need to be alert for increased distress on part of the client

Slide 31

Mental Health Assessment & Managing the Interview

- Assessment interview will likely take more time than with a neurotypical person
- Examiner needs to use language that correlates with the expressive and receptive language skills of the client
  - Simple language
  - Reflection
  - Stay away from abstract concepts and analogies

Slide 32

Mental Health Assessment & Managing the Interview

- Watch for signs the person is trying to respond to questions in a way that will please the interviewer.
- Parroting and perseverating habits may interfere with the accuracy of the responses.
- Multiple assessment interviews may be needed to obtain a full assessment.

Slide 33

Mental Health Assessment

I. Source of Information and Reason for Referral

II. History of Presenting Problem and Past Psychiatric History

III. Family Health History

IV. Social and Developmental History

Slide 34

Mental Health Assessment

I. Source of Information and Reason for Referral

- Who made the referral?
- What is different from baseline behavior?
- Why make the referral now?

Slide 35

Mental Health Assessment

II. History of Presenting Problem and Past Psychiatric History

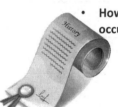

- How long has the problem occurred?
  - History of mental health treatment
  - Trauma history

Slide 36

Mental Health Assessment

III. Personal and Family Health History
- Medical, psychiatric, and substance abuse history
- Psychotropic medications
- Medical conditions
  - Genetic disorders
  - Hypo/hyper thyroid condition
  - Constipation
  - Epilepsy
  - Diabetes
  - Gastrointestinal problem

Slide 37

Mental Health Assessment

IV. Social/Developmental History

- Developmental milestones
- Relevant school history
- Work/vocational history
- Current work/vocational status
- Legal issues
- Relevant family dynamics
- Drug/alcohol history
- Abuse history (emotional/physical/sexual)
- Trauma history

Slide 38

Mental Health Assessment

Behavioral Status Review Reports

A. Recent Changes

B. Problem Behavior

C. Quality of Life Issues

Slide 39

Behavioral Status: Recent Changes: A

Name: _____ Today's Date: _____
Date of last appointment: _____ Person completing this form _____

A. Primary reason(s) for this consultation: _____
B. Life changes that have occurred within the last six (6) months

	Yes	No	Comments
1. Moves			
2. Deaths of significant others			
3. Staff or teacher changes			
4. New roommates/classmates			
5. Problems			
6. Loss of friend, pet, family member			
7. Loss of key staff/teacher			
8. Evidence of a delayed grief reaction			
9. Change in employment, program or leisure activities			

C. Acute medical problems or changes in past medical condition since last visit: _____

Slide 40

Behavioral Status:
Problem Behavior: B

	C	A	E	N/A	Comments
1. Is aggressive					
2. Is self injurious					
3. Appears anxious					
4. Socially isolates self					
5. Is overactive					
6. Is under-active					

Chronic: Person displays behavior on a daily basis, but severity may wax and wane
Acute: Behavior represents a dramatic change
Episodic: Periods of disturbance and periods of normal functioning
N/A: Non-Applicable

Slide 41

Behavioral Status:
Problem Behavior: B (continued)

	C	A	E	N/A	Comments
7. Engages in ritualistic behavior, compulsions					
8. Has self-stimulatory behavior					
9. Steals					
10. Has tantrums					
11. Is impulsive					
12. OTHER (explain):					

Chronic: Person displays behavior on a daily basis, but severity may wax and wane
Acute: Behavior represents a dramatic change
Episodic: Periods of disturbance and periods of normal functioning
N/A: Non-Applicable

Slide 42

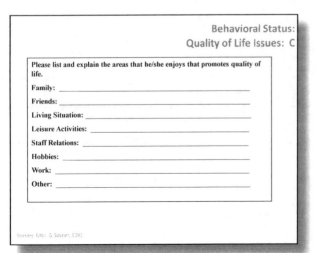

Behavioral Status:
Quality of Life Issues: C

Please list and explain the areas that he/she enjoys that promotes quality of life.
Family: _____
Friends: _____
Living Situation: _____
Leisure Activities: _____
Staff Relations: _____
Hobbies: _____
Work: _____
Other: _____

Slide 43

Minimal Data Collection

- Physical Health
- 24 Hour Sleep Data (month cycle)
- Medication Changes
- Eating Patterns
- Environmental Changes
- Mood Charting
  - Symptoms and Behavioral Management

Slide 44

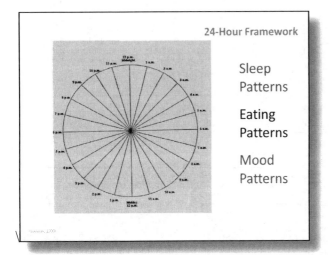

24-Hour Framework

Sleep Patterns

Eating Patterns

Mood Patterns

Slide 45

Exercise

Cal is a man with diagnoses of moderate intellectual disability and Autism Spectrum Disorder. He has a history of seizures, but is not currently treated for his seizure disorder and there are no seizures observed currently. A primary concern is that when he is in parking lots, he must search the entire lot to find any convertibles. If he is blocked from completing the search, he will become very aggressive and essentially do whatever it takes to do a thorough search regardless of the size of the lot. His family reports that they avoided any large parking lots while he lived at home. Numerous people have referred to this as OCD, though there is no formal diagnosis. There is an ongoing debate, at times bitter, between care providers, who consider this a symptom of ASD, and family who, consider this OCD.

Slide 46

Myth: Individuals with IDD Cannot Have a Verifiable Mental Health Disorder

PREMISE:
Maladaptive behaviors are a function of IDD

REALITY:
The full range of psychiatric disorders can be represented in persons with IDD

DIAGNOSTIC IMPLICATIONS:
Psychiatric diagnosis can be made using the DM-ID, DSM-5 records, service providers, family input, and client interview

Slide 47

Eight Diagnostic Principles For Recognizing Psychiatric Disorders In People with IDD

1. People with Intellectual/Developmental Disabilities suffer from the full range of psychiatric disorders.

2. Psychiatric disorders usually present as maladaptive behavior.

3. The origin of psychopathology has multiple etiologies.

Slide 48

Eight Diagnostic Principles For Recognizing Psychiatric Disorders In People with IDD (continued)

4. An acute psychiatric disorder may present as an exaggeration of longstanding maladaptive behavior

5. Maladaptive behavior rarely occurs alone

6. The severity of the problem is not diagnostically relevant

Slide 49

> **Eight Diagnostic Principles For Recognizing Psychiatric Disorders In People with IDD (continued)**
>
> 7. The clinical interview alone is rarely diagnostic.
>
> 8. It is very difficult to diagnose psychotic disorders in people with very limited verbal skills.
>
> Adapted from Sovner & Hurley, 1989

Slide 50

> **Barriers to Diagnosis and Treatment**
>
> **15 Complicating Diagnostic Factors**
>
> 1) Diagnostic Overshadowing
> 2) Problems with Poly pharmacy
> 3) Communication Deficits
> 4) Atypical Presentation of Psychiatric Disorders
> 5) Limited Life Experiences
> 6) Medical Conditions
> 7) Acquiescence
> 8) Learned Behavior
> 9) Aggression and SIB (self-injurious behavior)
> 10) Sensory Impairment
> 11) Behavioral Overshadowing
> 12) Medication Masking
> 13) Episodic Presentation
> 14) Division of Services
> 15) Lack of Expertise
>
> McGilivery & Sweetland, 2011

Slide 51

> **Barriers to Diagnosis and Treatment**
>
> **Complicating Diagnostic Factors (1-3)**
>
> 1) Diagnostic Overshadowing
>
> 2) Problems with Poly Pharmacy
>
> 3) Communication Deficits
>
> McGilivery & Sweetland, 2011

Slide 52

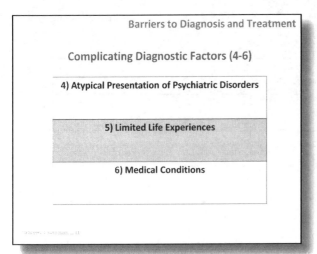

.Slide 53

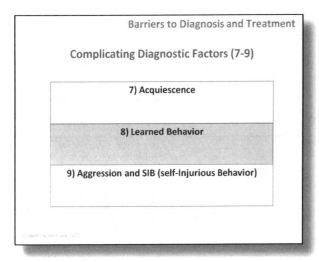

Slide 54

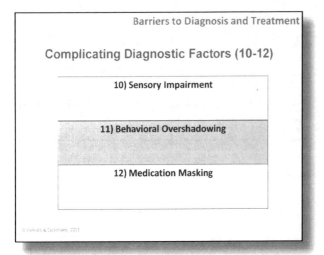

Slide 55

Barriers to Diagnosis and Treatment

Complicating Diagnostic Factors (13-15)

- 13) Episodic Presentation
- 14) Division of Services
- 15) Lack of Expertise

Slide 56

Psychiatric Symptoms/Learned Behaviors/Medication Conditions:

A Clinical Challenge

It can be difficult to distinguish whether a behavioral problem is associated with:

- A symptom of a psychiatric disorder
- A learned behavior
- A medical condition

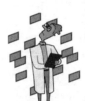

Slide 57

12 Indications that a Behavioral Pattern may be the result of a Psychiatric Condition

Slide 58

Assessment Considerations

Indications that a behavioral pattern may be the result of a psychiatric condition

1. The behavior occurs in all environments; it is not just exhibited in specific settings

2. Behavioral strategies have been largely ineffective

3. The individual doesn't appear to have control over their behavior. He/she doesn't appear to be able to start or stop the behavior at will.

Slide 59

Assessment Considerations

Indications that a behavioral pattern may be the result of a psychiatric condition

4. There are changes in sleep patterns; increased, decreased or disturbed sleep.

5. The individual is experiencing excessive mood or unusual mood patterns.

6. There are changes in the individual's appearance and a decline in their independent living skills.

Slide 60

Assessment Considerations

Indications that a behavioral pattern may be the result of a psychiatric condition

7. The person may start to engage in purposeful self-harm (cutting, hitting, scratching, pulling out hair).

8. The person may start to show signs of hallucination, such as staring to the side or corners and not appear to track conversations.

9. There may be changes in eating patterns such as eating less or more.

Slide 61

Assessment Considerations

Indications that a behavioral pattern may be the result of a psychiatric condition

10. The individual has a history of a psychiatric disorder that was in remission.

11. There is an acute onset of the behavior. If there is a particularly rapid onset with a significant change in mental status or cognitive functioning, rule out a possible delirium with an underlying medical cause.

12. There is an unusual change in behavior patterns, such as a significant change from baseline behavior

Slide 62

Medical Problems & Problem Behavior

- Why do medical causes of problem behaviors get missed?

- Why do we have to be.......
    Sherlock Holmes?

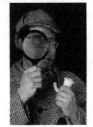

Slide 63

Medical Problems & Problem Behavior

Medical conditions can be present when behavioral problems are exhibited.

Medication effects / reactions can be present when behavioral problems are exhibited.

Medical conditions are often underdiagnosed.

Medical conditions can mask as behavioral problems.

Slide 64

Medical Problems & Problem Behavior

DRUG SIDE EFFECTS
Akathisia, Delirium, Dyskinesia
INFECTIONS
ENDOCRINOLOGICAL PROBLEMS
Thyroid problems   Diabetes
NEUROLOGICAL PROBLEMS
Epilepsy   Other movement problems
OTHER
Dental pain   Sleep apnea   Headaches
Hearing and vision problems   Back pain

Slide 65

Exercise

Each person to share information about a medication they know that has a relevant side effect.

Slide 66

Medical Problems & Problem Behavior

Medical Problems often under-recognized
Dental Problems often under-recognized

- Medical/Dental problems can cause SIB
- Need to identify if there is an underlying physical problem

Slide 67

Medical Problems & Problem Behavior

Case Example of Dental Pain & SIB

- 28 year old female with IDD referred to dental office for routine exam
- Mother noted that she began pulling out her hair
- Dental exam showed a fractured upper molar tooth, & tooth was extracted
- Mother subsequently reported that hair pulling ceased

Slide 68

Medical Problems & Problem Behavior

Condensed Medical Data in Chart

It is essential that all earlier medical data be available.

It is important that the past and present medical history be condensed in a format that can be easily read and placed in the person's chart.

Slide 69

Medical Problems & Problem Behavior

Medical Problems may cause significant alterations in mood and behavior that mimic acute psychiatric illness.

Slide 70

Medical Problems & Problem Behavior

Symptoms Reported by Informants:
Don't confuse phenomenology with etiology

- MANIA
  Irritable, restless, pacing, running back and forth, can't sit still, can't focus, can't get to sleep

- AKATHISIA
  Irritable, restless, pacing, running back and forth, can't sit still, can't focus, can't get to sleep

- DEPRESSION
  Crying, won't get out of bed, decreased concentration

- CONSTIPATION
  Crying, won't get out of bed, decreased concentration

Slide 71

Medical Problems & Problem Behavior

1. **Sleep Pattern**
   Quality and quantity of sleep can affect physical and mental health
   For example:
   a. Poor sleep ð fatigue ð irritability
   b. Depression ð poor sleep ð irritability
   c. Medical problem (discomfort caused by constipation) ð poor sleep ð irritability

   <u>Assessment Strategy</u>

   Maintain sleep data

Slide 72

Medical Problems & Problem Behavior

2. **Appetite Pattern**
   Changes in appetite can be clues in the assessment of mental health or physical problem

   Significant weight change may indicated a medical or mental health problems

   <u>Assessment Strategy</u>
   Monitor and document a person's weight on a weekly basis

Slide 73

Medical Problems & Problem Behavior

3. **Activity Level**
Activity level refers to the things a person usually does during the day. For example:
- going to work
- completing chores
- leisure time pursuits

Assessment Strategy
If a person's activity level changes drastically, it may be an unrecognized medical or mental health problem.

Slide 74

Medical Problems & Problem Behavior

3. **Activity Level (continued)**
Examples:

Arthritis ð decreased activity ð refuses to go to work ð could be viewed as non-compliant

Depression ð decreased activity ð refuses to go to work ð could be viewed as non-compliant

Slide 75

BEAMS

- Are there any changes in the current conditions?
- Are there any changes in:
  - B = behavior
  - E = energy level*
  - A = appetite
  - M = mood
  - S = sleep patterns
- How long the symptoms/changes have been occurring?
- Is there anything that appears to help the person feel better when these signs are present?
- In what context have these changes occurred?

MODULE II

ASSESSMENT PRACTICES

Post-Test

Module II: Integrated Assessment

___ 1. Which of the following is NOT an example of a medical condition that contributes to problem or maladaptive behavior?
    (a) Diabetes
    (b) Urinary tract infection
    (c) Acid reflux
    (d) None of the above

___ 2. Fill in the blank: The _____ of assessment considers the dynamic influence of four traditional models to arrive at a multi-modal assessment of maladaptive behavior that considers multiple determinants and how each may contribute to the function of behavior.
    (a) Communication Model
    (b) Behavior Model
    (c) Integrative Model
    (d) Medical Model

___ 3. Possible functions of challenging behavior in people with IDD/MI can include:
    (a) To gain attention from others.
    (b) To escape or avoid demands.
    (c) To obtain tangible items or opportunities
    (d) All of the above

___ 4. Best practice in assessment and diagnosis for people with IDD/MI refers to
    (a) The Bio-psychosocial model
    (b) Behavior analysis
    (c) Mental health assessments
    (d) An annual physical completed by a regulated health professional

___ 5. The bio-psychosocial model:
    (a) Incorporates the effects of biomedical and psychological factors and how these influences interrelate.
    (b) Does not require the review of existing data or background information to contribute to the assessment process.
    (c) Recognizes that clinical interview can be completed by reviewing the documented history and reports compiled about the person.
    (d) Recognizes that mental health is defined only by the relative absence of psychological distress.

___ 6. Which of the premises about people with an IDD is false?
   (a) The full range of psychiatric conditions expressed in the general population is also represented in persons with IDD.
   (b) Persons with IDD are considered to have a lower prevalence rate of MI than the general population.
   (c) Persons with an IDD may tell a clinician or care provider what he or she thinks they want to hear or agree to things to avoid the risk of disapproval.
   (d) None of the above.

___ 7. One of the first steps to completing a functional assessment is
   (a) Assessing the effectiveness of different approaches on the target behavior
   (b) Describing the target behavior; assigning an operational definition.
   (c) Identifying the patterns of triggers to help figure out how a behavior is maintained.
   (d) Understanding the behavior from the perspective of the person who directly observes it and the problem it causes for other people.

___ 8. The Integrative Model posits that
   (a) Problem behaviors can be completely attributed to the existence of a co-existing medical problem.
   (b) There are often multiple determinants that influence the expression of maladaptive behavior.
   (c) Manipulating the environment in such a way as to increase or decrease problem behavior assists in identifying the needs/emotions or a person with IDD.
   (d) The most effective treatment of problem behavior is teaching communication skills.

___ 9. Which of the following is the most suggestive indicator that a behavior pattern may be the result of a mental illness?
   (a) The behavior never occurs when the person's favorite direct support professional is supporting him/her.
   (b) The person appears to be able to start and stop the behavior at will.
   (c) The behavior is exhibited only at home.
   (d) The behavior occurs in all environments; it is not just observed in specific settings.

___ 10. Which one of the following statements is accurate?
   (a) Medical problems in people with IDD are easily recognized.
   (b) Dental problems in people with IDD are easily recognized.
   (c) Rapid onset in a change in behavior patterns is likely because behavioral problems are directly associated with having the condition of IDD.
   (d) Causes of SIB in people with IDD can be related to an underlying medical condition.

Module III

Mental Health Evaluations

Pre-Test

Module III: Mental Health Evaluations

___ 1. Which of the following is an effect of IDD in Clinical presentation?
   (a) Baseline exaggeration
   (b) Eltdown distortion
   (c) Integrative formations
   (d) Crohn's Disease

___ 2. What is the purpose of a Mental Status Exam?
   (a) To measure Intellectual Functioning
   (b) To determine immigration status
   (c) To create a snapshot of the mental status at the time of the assessment
   (d) To make an authoritative diagnosis of mental illness

___ 3. Which of the following is NOT considered in a Mental Status Exam?
   (a) Mood and affect
   (b) Yuggoth's six factors of disability
   (c) Appearance and behavior
   (d) Judgment and insight

___ 4. Who can complete a Mental Status Exam?
   (a) A parent
   (b) A regular education teacher
   (c) An attorney
   (d) A regulated health or mental health professional

___ 5. When might a Mental Status Exam best be performed?
   (a) At an emergency room during an intake
   (b) During an arrest
   (c) Upon being aroused from sedation
   (d) In the middle of a serious behavioral incident

___ 6. Which of the following is NOT a consideration around Intellectual Distortion as related to a Mental Status Exam?
   (a) Inability to label one's own experiences
   (b) Inability to understand common idioms
   (c) Inability to meet ISP goals
   (d) Difficulty describing psychological functioning to others

___ 7. Fill in the blank: Mental Status Exam often must be _____ for persons with IDD
   (a) Ignored
   (b) Modified
   (c) Diluted
   (d) Omitted

___ 8. In assessing General Appearance and Behavior in a Mental Status Exam, a reviewer would NOT consider:
   (a) Terrified facial expression
   (b) Refusal of participation in the interview
   (c) Use of pnakotic language
   (d) Excessive motor activity

___ 9. How might an examiner assess Mood and Affect to a Mental Status Exam?
   (a) Use of Pickman's Model
   (b) Asking the person to use faces to indicate emotions
   (c) Assessing range of motion
   (d) Hazred's Test

___ 10. In assessing Thought Process and Content during a Mental Status Exam, which of the following would least relevant?
   (a) Attire
   (b) Paranoid ideation
   (c) Phobias
   (d) Delusion

Slide 1

Module III

Mental Health Evaluation:
Mental Status Examinations
(MSE)

Slide 2

This module includes information about best practices in mental health evaluation for persons with IDD with a focus on mental status examination (MSE).

Slide 3

Learning Objectives

- Summarize the importance of assessing the cognitive developmental level of the person with IDD as it pertains to Mental Status Examination
- Describe three components of the Mental Status Examination
- Describe the 11 domains and how they are pertinent to the assessment process
- Describe how the developmental level of the person is related to the assessment process
- Articulate the purpose of the DSM and how it is used in the diagnostic process

Slide 4

Definitions

Affect: the observable expression of emotion

Psychomotor activity: movement or muscle activity related to mental processes

Thought process: brain processing information to form concepts, make decisions, reason, and problem solve

Cognitive functions: the mental processes involved in gaining knowledge and comprehension - thinking, knowing, remembering, judging, and problem-solving. These are higher-level functions of the brain and encompass language, imagination, perception, and planning.

Judgement: process by which people make decisions and form conclusions based on available information and material combined with thought and experience

Insight: self-understanding – the awareness of own attitudes, feelings, and behavior

Slide 5

Mental Health Evaluation

Effects of IDD in Clinical Presentation

The interaction between IDD and MI are a result of four factors that reflect the profound biopsychosocial affects of developmental disabilities

1. Intellectual Distortion
2. Psychosocial Masking
3. Cognitive Disintegration
4. Baseline Exaggeration

Slide 6

Mental Health Evaluation

Four Nonspecific Factors Associated with IDD That Influence the Diagnostic Process

Factor 1: Intellectual Distortion

<u>Definition</u>: Refers to the developmental effects of IDD on the person's diminished ability to think abstractly and communicate intelligibly

<u>Clinical Impact</u>: Inability for person to label his/her own experiences and report them

<u>Example</u>: When asked if he/she "hears voices", the person might respond "yes" without fully comprehending the implication of the question

Slide 7

Mental Health Evaluation

Four Nonspecific Factors Associated with IDD That Influence the Diagnostic Process

Factor 2: Psychosocial Masking

Definition: Impoverished social skills and life experiences can influence the content of psychiatric symptoms

Clinical Impact: The person with IDD might present significant symptomology that occurs within the developmental framework

Example: A person with moderate level of IDD, might believe he/she can drive a car and this can be a manifestation of grandiosity

Slide 8

Mental Health Evaluation

Four Nonspecific Factors Associated with IDD That Influence the Diagnostic Process

Factor 3: Cognitive Disintegration

Definition: Stress-induced disruption of information processing – Tendency of person with IDD to become disorganized under stress

Clinical Impact: Bizarre presentation and psychotic-like state may be misdiagnosed as schizophrenia

Example: Vulnerability to high levels of stress and overload of cognitive functioning may lead to atypical clinical presentation

Slide 9

Mental Health Evaluation

Four Nonspecific Factors Associated with IDD That Influence the Diagnostic Process

Factor 4: Baseline Exaggeration

Definition: Pre-existing maladaptive behaviors, that were not attributed to mental illness, may increase in frequency and intensity with the onset of a psychiatric disorder

Clinical Impact: Creates difficulty in establishing illness features, target symptoms, and outcome measures

Example: SIB (Self Injurious Behavior) or aggression, that occurred infrequently may suddenly increase in severity at onset of a psychiatric disorder

Slide 10

The Mental Status Exam

- The Mental Status Exam can only be administered by a regulated health or mental health professional such as a physician, nurse, psychologist or psychiatrist.

- A direct support professional can contribute to the process by being familiar with the components of the exam and the information they may need to assist the person to receive an accurate assessment.

Slide 11

Mental Status Examination (MSE)

- Systemic observation and recording about a person's thinking, emotions, and behavior
- MSE for people with IDD needs to be modified
- Useful way to organize and standardize the data of patient observation
- MSE is a snapshot of the mental status at the time of the assessment. The MSE can be used as a tool to note change in the status from one point-in-time to another.
- MSE is a diagnostic measurement. Data from care providers and patient history can be helpful.

Slide 12

Mental Status Examination (MSE)

I. General Appearance & Behavior
II. Mood and Affect
III. Psychomotor Activity and Speech
IV. Thought Process and Content
V. Cognitive Function
VI. Judgment and Insight

Slide 13

Mental Status Examination (MSE)

I. General Appearance & Behavior
- Assesses person's attentiveness and effective participation in interview
- Notes persons attitude toward examiner
- Assesses posture and general motor activity
- Notes facial expression
- Notes personal hygiene and grooming
- Assesses weight status

Note : All of the above is based on the cognitive developmental level of the individual with IDD.

Slide 14

Mental Status Examination (MSE)

I. General Appearance & Behavior (cont.)
- The clinician may need to rely on collateral information about the person's baseline appearance and behavior
- Baseline for a person with IDD may be very different from the neuro-typical person. For example, in a person with ASD, body posturing, self-hugging, and finger flicking may be the typical baseline behavior for a person on the Spectrum

Note : All of the above is based on the cognitive developmental level of the individual with IDD.

Slide 15

Exercise

Appearance in relation to …….
Body Build …..
Clothing Appropriate to…
Clean, neat, tidy, …..
Hygiene and grooming ….
Odor …
Facial expression ….
Eye Contact ….
Other things that are noteworthy……

Slide 16

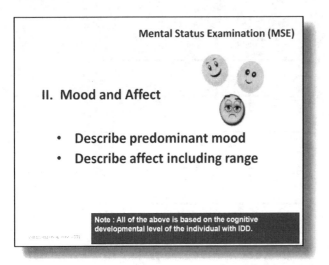

Slide 17

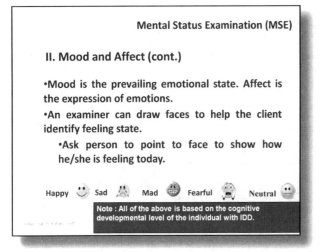

Slide 18

Exercise

II. Mood and affect

- Appropriateness of affect /Appropriate or inappropriate to situation. Congruous / Incongruous
- Range of affect ...
- Stability of affect ....
- Attitude during encounter ....
- Specific mood or feelings ....observed or reported
- Anxiety Level Rate .....

Slide 19

Mental Status Examination (MSE)

III. Psychomotor Activity and Speech
- Assesses psychomotor activity and notes
  - Rate of psychomotor activity (e.g., agitated, slowed)
  - Presence of abnormal movements
- Assesses speech and notes amount, volume, rate, organization of speech

Note: All of the above is based on the cognitive developmental level of the individual with IDD.

Slide 20

Mental Status Examination (MSE)

III. Psychomotor Activity and Speech (cont.)
- Examiner will need other collateral data in understanding the typical psychomotor activity and speech organization for the person.
  - For example, people who have Fragile X often have difficulty with gross motor coordination, which may lead to assessment as abnormal movements in absence of information about the effect of the syndrome.

Note: All of the above is based on the cognitive developmental level of the individual with IDD.

Slide 21

Exercise

III. Psychomotor Behavior
- Gait ...
- Handshake ...
- Abnormal movements ...
- Posture ....
- Rate of movements ...
- Co-ordination of

Slide 22

Mental Status Examination (MSE)

IV. Thought Process and Content
- Assess thought abnormalities
- Evaluate the content of thought
- Notes presence of delusions/ hallucinations (if so, what type of hallucinations)

Note: All of the above is based on the cognitive developmental level of the individual with IDD.

Slide 23

Mental Status Examination (MSE)

IV. Thought Process and Content (cont.)
- Clinical challenge in identifying abnormal thoughts and perceptions related to mental illness, compared to behaviors associated with the cognitive / developmental level of the individual
- Similarities between behaviors normal in young children without IDD and adults with IDD (i.e., self talk, imaginary friends, and rich fantasy life)

Note: All of the above is based on the cognitive developmental level of the individual with IDD.

Slide 24

Exercise

I. Thought Process
Clarity
Relevance / logic
Flow
Rapidly shifting ideas/thoughts?...
Perseveration ...
Pressure of speech ....
II. Content
Thoughts content consistent with reality?

Slide 25

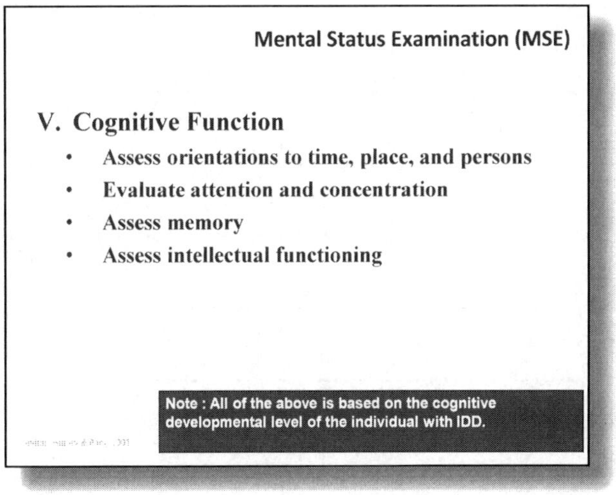

Mental Status Examination (MSE)

V. Cognitive Function
- Assess orientations to time, place, and persons
- Evaluate attention and concentration
- Assess memory
- Assess intellectual functioning

Note : All of the above is based on the cognitive developmental level of the individual with IDD.

Slide 26

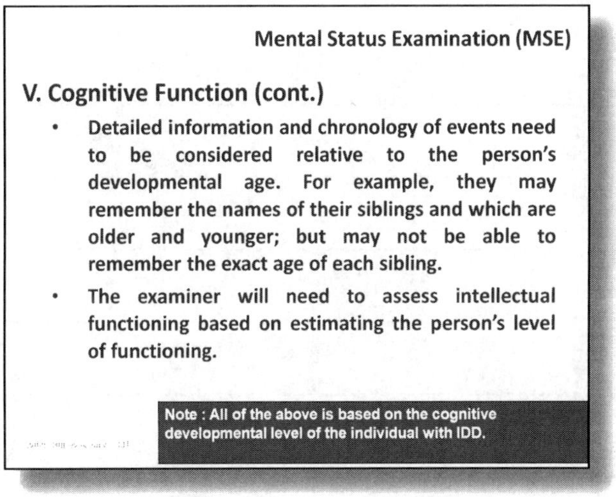

Mental Status Examination (MSE)

V. Cognitive Function (cont.)
- Detailed information and chronology of events need to be considered relative to the person's developmental age. For example, they may remember the names of their siblings and which are older and younger; but may not be able to remember the exact age of each sibling.
- The examiner will need to assess intellectual functioning based on estimating the person's level of functioning.

Note : All of the above is based on the cognitive developmental level of the individual with IDD.

Slide 27

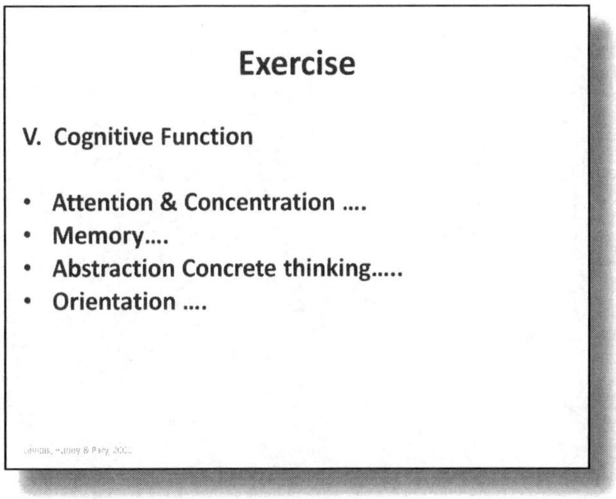

Exercise

V. Cognitive Function

- Attention & Concentration ….
- Memory….
- Abstraction Concrete thinking…..
- Orientation ….

Slide 28

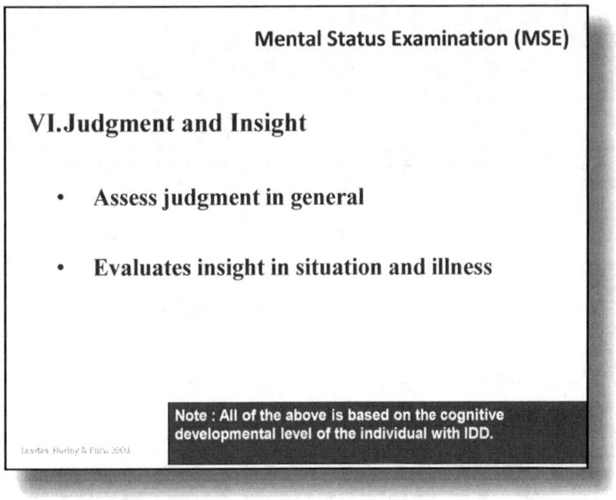

Mental Status Examination (MSE)

VI. Judgment and Insight

- Assess judgment in general
- Evaluates insight in situation and illness

Note: All of the above is based on the cognitive developmental level of the individual with IDD.

Slide 29

Exercise

VI. Judgement and Insight ….

Impulsive behavior ….
Insight into illness ….
Examples….

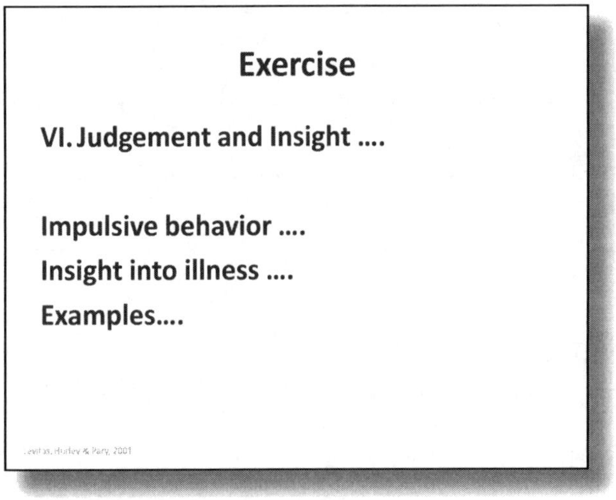

Post-Test

Module III: Mental Health Evaluations

___ 1. Which of the following is an effect of IDD in Clinical presentation?
    (a) Baseline exaggeration
    (b) Eltdown distortion
    (c) Integrative formations
    (d) Crohn's Disease

___ 2. What is the purpose of a Mental Status Exam?
    (a) To measure Intellectual Functioning
    (b) To determine immigration status
    (c) To create a snapshot of the mental status at the time of the assessment
    (d) To make an authoritative diagnosis of mental illness

___ 3. Which of the following is NOT considered in a Mental Status Exam?
    (a) Mood and affect
    (b) Yuggoth's six factors of disability
    (c) Appearance and behavior
    (d) Judgment and insight

___ 4. Who can complete a Mental Status Exam?
    (a) A parent
    (b) A regular education teacher
    (c) An attorney
    (d) A regulated health or mental health professional

___ 5. When might a Mental Status Exam best be performed?
    (a) At an emergency room during an intake
    (b) During an arrest
    (c) Upon being aroused from sedation
    (d) In the middle of a serious behavioral incident

___ 6. Which of the following is NOT a consideration around Intellectual Distortion as related to a Mental Status Exam?
    (a) Inability to label one's own experiences
    (b) Inability to understand common idioms
    (c) Inability to meet ISP goals
    (d) Difficulty describing psychological functioning to others

___ 7. Fill in the blank: Mental Status Exam often must be _____ for persons with IDD
(a) Ignored
(b) Modified
(c) Diluted
(d) Omitted

___ 8. In assessing General Appearance and Behavior in a Mental Status Exam, a reviewer would NOT consider:
(a) Terrified facial expression
(b) Refusal of participation in the interview
(c) Use of pnakotic language
(d) Excessive motor activity

___ 9. How might an examiner assess Mood and Affect to a Mental Status Exam?
(a) Use of Pickman's Model
(b) Asking the person to use faces to indicate emotions
(c) Assessing range of motion
(d) Hazred's Test

___ 10. In assessing Thought Process and Content during a Mental Status Exam, which of the following would least relevant?
(a) Attire
(b) Paranoid ideation
(c) Phobias
(d) Delusion

Module IV

Signs and Symptoms of Mental Illness

Pre-Test

Module IV – Signs and Symptoms of Mental Illness

___ 1. The prevalence of depression among adults with IDD is estimated to be:
   (a) Less than 1%.
   (b) 2%
   (c) 15%
   (d) 50%

___ 2. Which of the following is identified as a potential symptom of depression in someone with IDD?
   (a) Chronic constipation
   (b) Leaving tasks incomplete
   (c) No longer getting up for work/activities
   (d) None of the above

___ 3. Which of the following is false?
   (a) Bipolar disorder is the most common mental illness among people with IDD.
   (b) Borderline personality disorder is treatable.
   (c) Symptoms of mental illness may present differently among people with IDD.
   (d) All of the above

___ 4. Type of anxiety disorders listed in the DSM 5 include:
   (a) Panic disorder
   (b) Social anxiety disorder
   (c) Specific phobias
   (d) All of the above

___ 5. The DM ID is helpful because it:
   (a) It provides a comprehensive overview of the nature of IDD in general.
   (b) Includes information on presentation of different mental illness among people with IDD.
   (c) Gives the etiology of various mental illnesses
   (d) None of the above

___ 6. The DM ID offers which of the following in regards to self-mutilation among people with IDD?
   (a) It is always a symptom of Borderline Personality Disorder
   (b) It is not a symptom of Borderline Personality Disorder
   (c) It can be attributed to different causes
   (d) It does not occur frequently enough to be considered

___ 7. Which of the following is NOT a type of Personality Disorder listed in the DSM 5?
(a) General Personality Disorder
(b) Paranoid Personality Disorder
(c) Dependent Personality Disorder
(d) Cyclopean Personality Disorder

___ 8. Challenges with sleeping due to increased energy, inflated self-esteem, and disorganized speech and increase in vocalizations may be the presentation of Mania in individuals with IDD with a diagnosis of
(a) Borderline Personality Disorder
(b) Autism
(c) Bipolar Disorder
(d) Schizophrenia

___ 9. What differentiates the anxiety most people feel at different times in life (taking a test, going for a job interview) from anxiety disorders?
(a) Whether or not people have an intellectual disability
(b) The amount of impairment anxiety can cause to their everyday lives
(c) If it results in self injury such as skin picking or pinching
(d) There is no difference

___ 10. Ruling out medical conditions and considering that "self-talk" may be a learning tool/coping skill for people with IDD are important diagnostic concerns for which disorder?
(a) Depression
(b) Anxiety
(c) Personality Disorders
(d) Psychosis

Slide 1

Module IV

Signs and Symptoms of Mental Illness

Slide 2

This module includes information regarding Signs and Symptoms of Depressive Disorders, Bipolar Disorder, Anxiety Disorders, Personality Disorders, and Psychosis.

The module highlights the importance of observation and behavioral equivalence.

Slide 3

Learning Objectives

List three signs commonly present in people who have ID and the following diagnoses:
- Depression
- Bipolar Disorder
- Anxiety
- Personality Disorders
- Psychosis

Articulate the importance of observation in the assessment process.

Slide 4

DEPRESSION

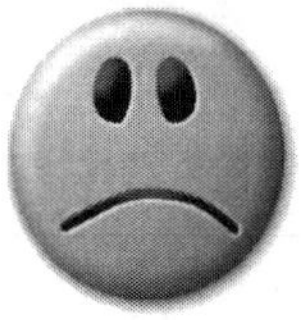

Slide 5

Depression

The prevalence of depression among adults with intellectual/developmental disability is estimated to be 2.2%.

Slide 6

Depression

- Can significantly disrupt school, work, family relationships, social life, etc.
- Onset tends to be more insidious and changes less dramatic (Deb et al., 2001)
- Increased prevalence in some symptoms as compared to typical population (Matson et al., 1988)
- Depression is among the most common psychiatric disorders in persons with IDD (Lamon & Reiss, 1987)

Slide 7

Depression

Public Figures who have/had Depression

- Abraham Lincoln, U.S. President
- Isaac Newton, Scientist
- Buzz Aldrin, Astronaut
- Terry Bradshaw, Former Quarterback
- Drew Carey, Actor/Comedian
- Leo Tolstoy, Author

Slide 8

Depression

DSM 5 Symptom for Depression	Presentation in Someone with IDD
DSM-5: Change in terminology to Major Depressive Disorder	• Frequent unexplained crying • Decrease in laughter and smiling • General irritability and subsequent aggression or self-injury • Sad facial expression
Markedly diminished interest or pleasure in all, or almost all, activities most of the day nearly every day	• No longer participates in favorite activities • Reinforcers no longer valued • Increased time spent alone • Refusals of most work/social activities

Slide 9

Depression

DSM 5 Symptom for Depression	Presentation in Someone with IDD
Weight Change/ Appetite Change	• Measured weight changes • Increased refusals to come to table to eat • Unusually disruptive at meal times • Constant food seeking behaviors
Insomnia	• Disruptive at bed time • Repeatedly gets up at night • Difficulty falling asleep • No longer gets up for work/activities • Early morning awakening
Hypersomnia	• Over 12 hours of sleep per day • Naps frequently

Slide 10

Depression

DSM 5 Symptom for Depression	Presentation in Someone with IDD
Psychomotor Agitation	• Restless, Fidgety, Pacing • Increased disruptive behavior
Psychomotor Retardation	• Sits for extended periods • Moves slowly • Takes longer than usual to complete activities

Slide 11

Depression

DSM 5 Symptom for Depression	Presentation in Someone with IDD
Fatigue/Loss of Energy	• Needs frequent breaks to complete simple activity • Slumped/tired body posture • Does not complete tasks with multiple steps
Inappropriate guilt	• Statements like "I'm dumb," "I'm retarded," etc. • Seeming to seek punishment • Social isolation

Slide 12

Depression

DSM 5 Symptom for Depression	Presentation in Someone with IDD
Lack of Concentration/ Diminished Ability to Think/Indecisiveness	• Decreased work output • Does not stay with tasks • Decrease in IQ upon retesting
Thoughts of Death	• Preoccupation with family member's death • Talking about committing or attempting suicide • Fascination with violent movies/television shows

Slide 13

Treatment Strategies (Depression)

- Psychotherapy (individual and/or group)
- Regular exercise
- Antidepressant medication
- Regular scheduling of pleasurable activities
- Learning stress management strategies
- Social skill training
- Positive environment and support strategies

Slide 14

What symptoms of depression might look like for a person with IDD...

Set Up:	Set Off:	So I:	And I get or avoid:
Depression Not that interested in work.	Cued regarding going to work	Ignore the cue and become aggressive	Avoid going to work. Work and paycheck used to be an incentive, but due to depression, formerly preferred events are no longer preferred.

Slide 15

BIPOLAR DISORDER

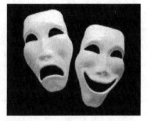

Slide 16

Bipolar Disorder

- **Causes mood swings**
- Persons with Bipolar Disorder may have periods of mania and periods of depression as well as normal moods.
- The length of cycle between moods can vary between rapid cycling or more slowly over time.
- Only a minority of people alternate back and forth between mania and depression with each cycle; in most, one or the other predominates to some extent. (Beers & Berkow, 1999)
- During a manic episode, a person will display oversupply of confidence and energy

Slide 17

Bipolar Disorder

Public Figures who have/had Bipolar Disorder

- Carrie Fisher, Actor/Author
- Linda Hamilton, Actor
- Catherine Zeta Jones, Actor
- Vincent Van Gogh, Artist (suspected)
- Jane Pauley, Journalist
- Sting, Musician
- Ludwig van Beethoven, Composer/Musician (suspected)

Slide 18

Bipolar Disorder

DSM 5 Symptoms of Mania	Presentation in Someone with IDD
Elevated, expansive, or irritable mood and abnormally and persistently increasing goal-directed activity or energy	• Smiling, hugging or being affectionate with people who previously were not favored by the individual • **Boisterousness** • Over-reactivity to small incidents • **Extreme excitement** • Excessive laughing and giggling • **Self-injury associated with irritability** • Enthusiastic greeting of everyone

Slide 19

Bipolar Disorder

DSM 5 Symptoms of Mania	Presentation in Someone with IDD
Increased energy or activity and 3 or more of the following: Inflated self-esteem/grandiosity; Decreased need for sleep; More talkative/pressured speech; Flight of ideas; Distractibility; Increase in psychomotor agitation; Excessive involvement in activities that have a high potential for painful consequences	• Behavioral challenges when prompted to go to try to sleep • Constantly getting up at night • Seems rested after not sleeping (i.e., not irritable due to lack of sleep as is common in depression)

Slide 20

DSM 5 Symptoms of Mania	Presentation in Someone with IDD
Inflated Self-esteem/ Grandiosity	• Making improbable claims (e.g., is a staff member, has mastered all necessary skills, etc.) • Dramatic physical presentation • Dressing provocatively • Demanding rewards
Flight of Ideas	• Disorganized speech • Thoughts not connected • Quickly changing subjects

Slide 21

Bipolar Disorder

DSM 5 Symptoms of Mania	Presentation in Someone with IDD
More Talkative/ Pressured Speech	• Increased singing • Increased swearing • Perseverative speech • Screaming • Frequent interrupting • Non-verbal communication increases • Increase in vocalizations

Slide 22

Bipolar Disorder

DSM 5 Symptoms of Mania	Presentation in Someone with IDD
Distractibility	• Decrease in work/task performance • Leaving tasks incomplete • Inability to settle (e.g., stay seated and focus on favorite TV show, stay seated through a complete activity when generally able to do so)

Slide 23

Bipolar Disorder

DSM 5 Symptoms of Mania	Presentation in Someone with IDD
Agitation/Increase in Goal Directed Behavior	• Pacing • Negativism • Working on many activities at once • Fidgeting • Aggression • Rarely sits
Excessive Pleasurable Activities	• Increase in masturbation • Giving away/spending money

Slide 24

Bipolar Disorder

Treatment Strategies

- Psychotherapy with a focus on understanding and managing the disorder

- Environmental and social modification (i.e., increase supervision to ensure safety)

- Positive support strategies

- Mood stabilizing and antidepressant medication

Slide 25

What symptoms of bi-polar disorder might look like for a person with IDD...

Set Up:	Set Off:	So I:	And I get or avoid:
Bi-polar cycling into manic phase	Want to continue activity for many hours into the night	I begin to scream and wake up the rest of the house	Staff allow me to return to activity since it is quieter than my screaming.
Not always a good sleeper			
Not a lot of friends	Staff interrupt the activity		

Slide 26

Anxiety Disorders

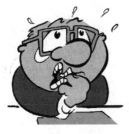

Slide 27

Anxiety Disorders

Anxiety Disorders include a large number of conditions characterized by:
- Sense of apprehension
- Physiological symptoms – sweating, increased heart rate, increased rate of respiration
- Restlessness, fatigue, irritability, sleep disturbances, difficulty concentrating, muscle tension, personality changes.
- Lack of cause or situation does not warrant the extent of the reaction.

Slide 28

Anxiety Disorders

Public Figures who have/had Anxiety Disorders

- Barbara Streisand, Singer/Actor/Director
- Nikola Tesla, Scientist/Inventor
- Charles Darwin, Naturalist/Author
- Johnny Depp, Actor
- Neil Young, Musician

Slide 29

Types of Anxiety Disorders

Among the anxiety disorders listed in the DSM 5 are;
- **Specific phobias:** Marked fear or anxiety about specific objects or situations, such as snakes, heights, flying, etc.
- **Social anxiety disorder:** Marked fear or anxiety about one or more social situations in which the person is exposed to possible scrutiny by others.
- **Panic Disorder:** Recurrent, unexpected panic attacks.
- **Generalized anxiety disorder:** This disorder involves excessive, anxiety or worry occurring more days than not for at least 6 months, about a number of events or activities.

DSM 5, 2013

Slide 30

Anxiety Disorders

DSM 5 Symptoms of Generalized Anxiety Disorder	Presentation in Someone with IDD
A. Developmentally inappropriate and excessive fear or anxiety . Anxiety or worry associated with 3 or more of the following 6: · Restlessness · Easily fatigued · Difficulty concentrating · Irritability · Muscle tension · Sleep disturbances	• No adaptation from criteria in DSM 5

Slide 31

Anxiety Disorders

DSM 5 Symptoms of Generalized Anxiety Disorder	Presentation in Someone with IDD
B. Fear, anxiety or avoidance is persistent, lasting at least 4 wks	• Inapplicable in persons with Profound IDD (may mean it's diagnosis is not possible based on the person's limited ability for insight about thoughts or articulate thoughts and feelings).
C. Focus of Anxiety or worry	• No adaptation from DSM 5 for mild to moderate IDD. Difficulty to apply in persons with severe IDD. Inapplicable in persons with profound IDD.

Slide 32

Anxiety Disorders

DSM 5 Symptoms of Generalized Anxiety Disorder	Presentation in Someone with IDD
E. Anxiety or worry causes clinically significant distress or impairment in social, academic, occupational, or other important areas of functioning.	• No adaptation from DSM 5
F. Anxiety or worry is not connected to the physiological effects of a substance, e.g., medication, drug or medical condition or not better explained by another disorder	• No adaptation from DSM 5

Slide 33

Anxiety Disorders

Treatment Strategies

- **Psychotherapy with a focus on understanding and managing the disorder**
- Environmental and social modification
- **Social skill training**
- Regular exercise
- **Wellness based approaches**
- Learning stress management strategies
- **Anti-anxiety medication**

Slide 34

What symptoms of anxiety might look like for a person with IDD…

Set Up:	Set Off:	So I:	And I get or avoid:
Person has an Anxiety Disorder and an Autism Spectrum Disorder	Family member interrupts routine	Begin to strip off my clothing	I am allowed to return to the routine I am comfortable following
Low tolerance for frustration			
History of conflict with family			
Bullying type of personality			

Slide 35

Personality Disorders

Slide 36

Personality Disorders

Personality Disorders are mental health disorders which cause difficulty perceiving and relating to situations and people including self. They are characterized by:
- **Rigid and unhealthy patterns of thinking and behaving across situations.**
- Frequent mood swings
- **Stormy relationships**
- Social isolation
- **Angry outbursts**
- Suspicion and mistrust of others
- **Difficulty making friends**
- A need for instant gratification
- **Poor impulse control**
- Alcohol or substance abuse

Slide 37

Personality Disorders

Public Figures who have/had Personality Disorders

- Doug Ferrari – Comedian
- Herschel Walker, NFL Player/Heisman Trophy Winner

Slide 38

Types of Personality Disorders

Among the different types of Personality Disorders listed in the DSM 5 are:

- **General Personality Disorder:** Enduring pattern of inner thoughts or behavior that deviates markedly from the expectations of the individual's culture
- **Paranoid Personality Disorder:** Pervasive distrust or suspiciousness of others such that their behavior is interpreted as malevolent
- **Dependent Personality Disorder:** Pervasive and excessive need to be taken care of that leads to submissive and clinging behavior and fear of separation

Slide 39

Personality Disorders

DSM 5 Symptoms of Borderline Personality Disorder (indicated by 5 or more of the following)	Presentation in Someone with IDD
1) Frantic efforts to avoid real or imagined abandonment.	More reliant on caregivers than general population. Cultural sensitivities must also be considered.
2) Pattern of unstable and intense interpersonal relationships alternating between idealization and devaluation.	No adaptation from DSM 5

Slide 40

Personality Disorders

DSM 5 Symptoms of Borderline Personality Disorder	Presentation in Someone with IDD
3) Identity disturbance: markedly and persistently unstable self-image or sense of self.	• No adaptation – but note that expressions of self-image require fairly sophisticated verbal skills that may not be present in a person with IDD.
4) Impulsivity in at least 2 areas that are potentially self-damaging	• No adaptation from DSM-5 • Examples, spending, sexual activity, substance abuse, binge eating

Slide 41

Personality Disorders

DSM 5 Symptoms of Borderline Personality Disorder	Presentation in Someone with IDD
5) Recurrent suicidal behavior, gestures, threats, or self-mutilating behavior	• No adaptation but note that self-injury can be a frequent problem for people with IDD and can be attributed to different causes.
6) Mood reactivity causing attentive instability.	• No adaptation from DSM 5 • e.g., irritability, intense episodic dysphoria/feeling of unease, anxiety usually lasting only a few hours

Slide 42

Personality Disorders

DSM 5 Symptoms of Borderline Personality Disorder	Presentation in Someone with IDD
7) Chronic feelings of emptiness	• No adaptation - but note that expressions of feelings can require fairly sophisticated verbal skills that may not be present in a person with IDD
8) Inappropriate intense anger or difficulty controlling anger	• No adaptation – but note that anger problems are frequently noted for people with IDD.
9) Temporary paranoia brought on by stress or severe symptoms of dissociation	• No adaptation from DSM 5

Slide 43

Personality Disorders

Treatment Strategies
- Individual or group therapy – cognitive and dialectic behavior therapy are most effective
- Environmental and social modification
- Social skill training
- Regular exercise
- Positive Behavioral Supports
- Psychotropic medication can be helpful for primary presenting symptoms.
- Emotional regulation
- Learning stress management strategies/stress tolerance
- Positive identity development

Hughes 2008

Slide 44

What symptoms of Borderline Personality Disorder might look like for a person with IDD…

Set Up:	Set Off:	So I:	And I get or avoid:
Borderline Personality Disorder	Staff are arguing back and forth	Make the divide between staff bigger escalating their argument.	I get to watch the conflict and drama that result.
Lots of staff turnover			
Placed with people who are lower functioning Wants to "be" staff			
New manager creates conflict on the team			

Slide 45

Schizophrenia and other Psychosis

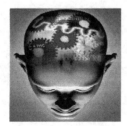

Slide 46

Psychosis

- The defining characteristics of psychosis are delusions, hallucinations, and disorganized speech or behavior.

- There is evidence that current diagnostic criteria from DSM 5 can be used reliably for people with IDD but behavioral disturbances do seem more significant for people with Severe to Profound IDD than with Mild IDD.

Slide 47

Psychosis

Public Figures who have/had Psychosis

- John Forbes Nash, Mathematician
- Lionel Aldridge, NFL Player (Super Bowl champion)
- Peter Green, Blues Musician/Founder Fleetwood Mac
- Jack Kerouac, Author
- Zelda Sayre Fitzgerald, American Novelist

Slide 48

Types of Psychosis

Among the Psychotic Disorders listed in the DSM 5 are;

- Schizoaffective Disorder
- Delusional Disorder
- Schizophreniform Disorder
- Substance/Medication Induced Psychotic Disorder

Slide 49

Psychosis

DSM 5 Symptoms Of Schizophrenia	Presentation in Someone with IDD
A) Two or more of the following present for a significant portion of a 1 month period: · Delusions · Hallucinations · Disorganized speech · Grossly disorganized behavior · Negative symptoms, i.e., affect flattening, newly evidenced inability to speak, general lack of motivation or desire to pursue meaningful goals.	• No adaptation – note that developmentally appropriate self-talk, imaginary friends, fantasy play, and beliefs based on faulty learning can be confused with hallucinations and delusions.

Slide 50

Psychosis

DSM 5 Symptoms of Schizophrenia	Presentation in Someone with IDD
B. Level of functioning in one or more major areas, such as work, interpersonal relations, or self-care is markedly below the level achieved prior to onset	• No Adaptation – but note that functional areas are dependent upon functioning level for the person.
C. Duration – continuous signs of the disturbance exist for at least six months.	• No adaptation from DSM 5 level of skill markedly below level achieved prior to onset for example, self-care skills, interpersonal relations,

Slide 51

Psychosis

DSM IV-TR Symptoms of Schizophrenia	Presentation in Someone with ID
D) Schizoaffective disorder and depressive bipolar disorder with psychotic features have been ruled out	• No adaptation from DSM-5
E) The disturbance is not due to direct physiological effects of substance or general medical condition	• No adaptation from DSM-5

Slide 52

Psychosis

DSM 5 Symptoms Of Schizophrenia	Presentation in Someone with IDD
F. If there is a history of Autism Spectrum Disorder or a Communication Disorder of childhood onset, the additional diagnosis of schizophrenia is made only if prominent delusions or hallucinations, in addition to other required symptoms of schizophrenia, are also present for at least one month	• No adaptation from DSM 5

Slide 53

Psychosis

Treatment Strategies

- Adhering to a daily routine
- **Social skill training**
- Vocational Training
- **Positive Support Strategies**
- Education regarding schizophrenia
- **Recreation Therapy**
- Antipsychotic medication

Slide 54

What symptoms of Psychosis might look like for a person with IDD...

Set Up:	Set Off:	So I:	And I get or avoid:
Psychosis Lives with 3 other people with IDD	Auditory hallucination at breakfast	Yell back to "the voice"	Roommates take their coffee out to the porch

Post-Test

Module IV – Signs and Symptoms of Mental Illness

___ 1. The prevalence of depression among adults with IDD is estimated to be:
   (a) Less than 1%.
   (b) 2%
   (c) 15%
   (d) 50%

___ 2. Which of the following is identified as a potential symptom of depression in someone with IDD?
   (a) Chronic constipation
   (b) Leaving tasks incomplete
   (c) No longer getting up for work/activities
   (d) None of the above

___ 3. Which of the following is false?
   (a) Bipolar disorder is the most common mental illness among people with IDD.
   (b) Borderline personality disorder is treatable.
   (c) Symptoms of mental illness may present differently among people with IDD.
   (d) All of the above

___ 4. Type of anxiety disorders listed in the DSM 5 include:
   (a) Panic disorder
   (b) Social anxiety disorder
   (c) Specific phobias
   (d) All of the above

___ 5. The DM ID is helpful because it:
   (a) It provides a comprehensive overview of the nature of IDD in general.
   (b) Includes information on presentation of different mental illness among people with IDD.
   (c) Gives the etiology of various mental illnesses
   (d) None of the above

___ 6. The DM ID offers which of the following in regards to self-mutilation among people with IDD?
   (a) It is always a symptom of Borderline Personality Disorder
   (b) It is not a symptom of Borderline Personality Disorder
   (c) It can be attributed to different causes
   (d) It does not occur frequently enough to be considered

___ 7. Which of the following is NOT a type of Personality Disorder listed in the DSM 5?
(a) General Personality Disorder
(b) Paranoid Personality Disorder
(c) Dependent Personality Disorder
(d) Cyclopean Personality Disorder

___ 8. Challenges with sleeping due to increased energy, inflated self-esteem, and disorganized speech and increase in vocalizations may be the presentation of Mania in individuals with IDD with a diagnosis of
(a) Borderline Personality Disorder
(b) Autism
(c) Bipolar Disorder
(d) Schizophrenia

___ 9. What differentiates the anxiety most people feel at different times in life (taking a test, going for a job interview) from anxiety disorders?
(a) Whether or not people have an intellectual disability
(b) The amount of impairment anxiety can cause to their everyday lives
(c) If it results in self injury such as skin picking or pinching
(d) There is no difference

___ 10. Ruling out medical conditions and considering that "self-talk" may be a learning tool/coping skill for people with IDD are important diagnostic concerns for which disorder?
(a) Depression
(b) Anxiety
(c) Personality Disorders
(d) Psychosis

Module V

From the DM-ID
to the
DM-ID-2

Pre-Test

Module V: From DM-ID to DM-ID-2

___ 1. The DM-ID is _____.
   (a) An acronym to describe people with ID
   (b) An organization concerning people with disabilities
   (c) A diagnostic manual for people with disabilities
   (d) A history book on people with ID

___ 2. The DM-ID diagnostic system _____.
   (a) Focuses on the International Classification System (ICD)
   (b) Focuses on comparing the DSM and the ICD diagnostic criteria.
   (c) Compares the DSM-5 and DM-ID-2 diagnostic criteria.
   (d) All of the above.

___ 3. _____ refers to the process of over-attributing an individual's symptoms to a particular condition.
   (a) Slanted condition
   (b) Aspect concentration
   (c) Diagnostic overshadowing
   (d) Specific review

___ 4. A(n) _____ perspective is emphasized throughout the DM-ID to assist the clinician in recognizing psychiatric disorders.
   (a) Developmental
   (b) Reactive
   (c) Aggregation
   (d) Disclosed

___ 5. Psychiatric diagnosis and treatment tends to
   (a) Require a blood test
   (b) Differ only by gender
   (c) Be consistent.
   (d) Vary greatly from person to person

___ 6. Which of the following is NOT a change a clinician should make when speaking to an individual with an intellectual disability?
   (a) Ask one simple question at a time
   (b) Wait for the answer before proceeding
   (c) Use music to soothe the individual
   (d) Use visuals

___ 7. In the assessment process, information on individuals with intellectual disabilities should be provided by:
   (a) Multiple sources of information
   (b) Strictly family
   (c) Clinicians/staff only
   (d) Only by the individual

___ 8. _____ denotes a set of behaviors that are genetically determined and are associated with a particular genetic disorder
   (a) Diagnostic overshadowing
   (b) Assessment procedure
   (c) Behavioral phenotype
   (d) Category

___ 9. A particular psychiatric disorder may be manifested differently between:
   (a) Men and woman
   (b) Different seasons
   (c) Different levels of disability (mild/moderate vs. severe/profound)
   (d) Different income levels

___ 10. Explanatory notes are based on
   (a) Helping doctors keep track of patients
   (b) Breaking down disorders for families to understand
   (c) Separating care providers from staff
   (d) Specific behavior characteristics in persons with IDD

Slide 1

> # Module V
>
> From the DM-ID
> To the
> DM-ID-2

Slide 2

> This module contains information about the DM-ID and the DM-ID-2 and how they assist in the diagnostic process for persons with IDD.

Slide 3

> ### Learning Objectives
> - Describe the purpose of the DM-ID-2
> - Identify 3 types of modifications of the DSM criteria which are contained in the DM-ID-2
> - Describe the significance of the cognitive developmental level in relationship to criteria subsets
> - Articulate why the DSM system does not apply to people who have language deficits

Slide 4

Limitations of DSM System

- **Diagnostic Overshadowing (Reiss, et al, 1982)**
- **Applicability of established diagnostic systems is increasingly suspect as the severity of IDD increases (Rush & Frances, 2000)**
- **DSM System relies on self report of signs and symptoms (DSM-IV-TR, DSM-5)**

Slide 5

DM–ID
Diagnostic Manual – Intellectual Disabilities

Developed By
National Association for the Dually Diagnosed
(NADD)
In association with
American Psychiatric Association
(APA)

Partial Funding from the Joseph P. Kennedy, Jr. Foundation
Published by the NADD Press, 2007

Slide 6

DM–ID: Two Manuals

Diagnostic Manual – Intellectual Disability: A Textbook of Diagnosis of Mental Disorders in Persons with Intellectual Disability

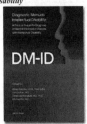

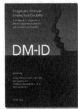

Diagnostic Manual – Intellectual Disability: A Clinical Guide for Diagnosis of Mental Disorders in Persons with Intellectual Disability

Slide 7

Description of DM-ID

- An adaptation to the *DSM-IV-TR*
- Designed to facilitate a more accurate psychiatric diagnosis
- Based on Expert Consensus Model
- Covers all major diagnostic categories as defined in *DSM-IV-TR*

Slide 8

Description of DM-ID (continued)

- Provides information to help with diagnostic process
- Addresses pathoplastic effect of IDD on psychopathology (how the disorder is manifested in people with IDD)
- Designed with a developmental perspective to help clinicians to recognize symptom profiles in adults and children with IDD

Slide 9

Description of DM-ID (continued)

- Empirically-based approach to identify specific psychiatric disorders in persons with IDD
- Provides state-of-the-art information about mental disorders in persons with IDD
- Provides adaptations of criteria, where appropriate

Slide 10

Field Study of the Clinical Usefulness of the DM-ID

Table 1: Clinician Impressions by Level of Intellectual Disability (%YES)

Item	Mild N=305	Moderate N=237	Severe/Profound N=285
Was the DM-ID easy to use (user friendly)?	72.4	68.6	62.6
Did you find the DM-ID clinically useful in the diagnosis of this patient?	74.9	67.8	66.0
Did DM-ID allow you to arrive at an appropriate psychiatric diagnosis for this patient?	85.6	83.3	80.2
Did DM-ID allow you to come up with a more specific diagnosis than you would have with the *DSM-IV-TR*?	36.1	38.0	35.9
Did DM-ID help you avoid using the NOS category?	63.2	63.3	54.9

Slide 11

The Publication of the DSM-5 Necessitates Revision of the DM-ID

THE DM-ID-2

Slide 12

DM-ID-2
Two Special Added-Value Chapters

- Assessment and Diagnostic Procedures

- Behavioral Phenotype of Genetic Disorders

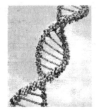

Slide 13

Assessment and Diagnostic Procedures Chapter

Psychiatric diagnosis is a challenge

Need to rely on multiple sources for information

Need to understand their challenges

Be empathetic

Slide 14

DM-ID-2 Assessment and Diagnostic Procedures Chapter

Special Considerations
- Use language that can be understood
- Confirm understanding

Establishing Chief Complaint and History
- Ask client
- Ask other individuals
- Obtain historical information

Slide 15

DM-ID-2 Assessment and Diagnostic Procedures Chapter

Historical Information

Slide 16

Behavioral Phenotype of Genetic Disorders Chapter

- Angelman Syndrome
- Chromosome 15q112-131 Duplication Syndrome
- Down Syndrome
- Fetal Alcohol Syndrome
- Fragile-X Syndrome
- Phenylketonuria
- Prader-Willi Syndrome
- Rubenstein-Taybi Syndrome
- Smith-Magenis Syndrome
- Tuberous Sclerosis Complex
- Velocardiofacial Syndrome
- Williams Syndrome

Slide 17

DM-ID-2
Behavioral Phenotype of Genetic Disorders Chapter
Phenotype and Behavioral Phenotype for Down Syndrome

Phenotype		Small head, mouth; upward slant to eyes; epicanthal folds; broad neck; hypothyroidism; hearing loss; visual impairments; cardiac problems; gastro-intestinal; orthopedic, and skin disorders; obesity
Behavioral Phenotype	Childhood	Oppositional and defiant; attention-deficit/hyperactivity disorder (ADHD); social, charming personality "stereotype"; self-talk
	Adulthood	Depressive disorders; obsessive-compulsive disorder; other anxiety disorders; dementia of the Alzheimer's type; mental disorders associated with hypothyroidism; atypical psychoses; self-talk

Slide 18

DM-ID-2
Diagnostic Chapter Structure

- **Review of Diagnostic Criteria**
  - **General description of the disorder**
  - **Summary of *DSM-5* criteria**

- Issues related to diagnosis in people with IDD

- **Review of Literature/Research**
  - **Evaluating level of evidence**

Slide 19

Application of Diagnostic Criteria to People with IDD

- General considerations
- **Adults with Mild to Moderate IDD**
- Adults with Severe or Profound IDD
- **Children and adolescents with IDD**

DM-ID-2

Slide 20

Etiology and Pathogenesis

- Risk Factors
  - **Biological Factors**
  - **Psychological Factors**
  - **Genetic Syndromes**

DM-ID-2 (continued)

Slide 21

Diagnostic Criteria

DSM-IV-TR Criteria	Applying Criteria to Mild-Moderate IDD	Applying Criteria to Severe-Profound IDD

DM-ID-2 (continued)

Slide 22

Diagnostic Criteria

DSM-IV-TR Criteria	Applying Criteria for IDD (Mild to Profound)

Slide 23

Modifications of the DSM-5 Criteria

1. Addition of symptom equivalents
2. Omission of symptoms
3. Changes in symptom count
4. Modification of symptom duration

Slide 24

Modifications of the DSM-5 Criteria

5. Modification of age requirements
6. Addition of explanatory notes
7. Criteria Sets that do not apply

Slide 25

Modification of *DSM-5* Criteria
Change in Count and Symptom Equivalent
Major Depressive Disorder

DSM-5 Criteria	Applying Criteria for Mild to Profound IDD
A. Five or more of the following symptoms have been present during the same 2 week period and represent a change from previous functioning. At least one of the symptoms is either (1) depressed mood or (2) loss of interest or pleasure.	A. Four or more symptoms have been present during the same 2 week period and represent a change from previous functioning. At least one of the symptoms is either (1) depressed mood or (2) loss of interest or pleasure or (3) irritable mood

Slide 26

Modifications of *DSM-5* Criteria
Modification of Age
Antisocial Personality Disorder

DSM-5 Criteria	Applying Criteria for Individuals with IDD
A. There is a pervasive pattern of disregard for and violation of the rights of others occurring since age 15 years, as indicated by three (or more) of the following:	A. There is a pervasive pattern of disregard for and violation of the rights of others occurring since age 18 years, as indicated by three (or more) of the following:
B. The individual is at least age 18 years	B. The individual is at least age 21 years
C. There is evidence of Conduct Disorder with the onset before age 15 years	C. There is evidence of Conduct Disorder with onset before age 18 years

Slide 27

Modification of Criteria
Addition of Explanatory Note
Manic Episode

DSM-IV-TR Criteria	Applying Criteria for Mild to Profound IDD
A. A distinct period of abnormally persistently elevated, expansive or irritable mood, lasting at least 1 week (or any duration if hospitalization is necessary)	A. No adaptation. Note: Observers may report that the individual with IDD: *has loud inappropriate laughing or singing, is excessively giddy or silly; is intrusive, getting into other's space; and smiles excessively and in ways that are not appropriate to the social context. Elated mood may be alternating with irritable mood*

Slide 28

The Future

DM-ID 2

In Development

Edited By:
Robert Fletcher, DSW, ACSW, NADD-CC
Jarrett Barnhill, M.D., DFAPA, FAACAP
Sally Ann Cooper, BSc (Hons), MB, BS, MD, FRCPsych

Post-Test

Module V: From DM-ID to DM-ID-2

___ 1. The DM-ID is _____.
   (a) An acronym to describe people with ID
   (b) An organization concerning people with disabilities
   (c) A diagnostic manual for people with disabilities
   (d) A history book on people with ID

___ 2. The DM-ID diagnostic system _____.
   (a) Focuses on the International Classification System (ICD)
   (b) Focuses on comparing the DSM and the ICD diagnostic criteria.
   (c) Compares the DSM-5 and DM-ID-2 diagnostic criteria.
   (d) All of the above.

___ 3. _____ refers to the process of over-attributing an individual's symptoms to a particular condition.
   (a) Slanted condition
   (b) Aspect concentration
   (c) Diagnostic overshadowing
   (d) Specific review

___ 4. A(n) _____ perspective is emphasized throughout the DM-ID to assist the clinician in recognizing psychiatric disorders.
   (a) Developmental
   (b) Reactive
   (c) Aggregation
   (d) Disclosed

___ 5. Psychiatric diagnosis and treatment tends to
   (a) Require a blood test
   (b) Differ only by gender
   (c) Be consistent.
   (d) Vary greatly from person to person

___ 6. Which of the following is <u>NOT</u> a change a clinician should make when speaking to an individual with an intellectual disability?
   (a) Ask one simple question at a time
   (b) Wait for the answer before proceeding
   (c) Use music to soothe the individual
   (d) Use visuals

___ 7. In the assessment process, information on individuals with intellectual disabilities should be provided by:
(a) Multiple sources of information
(b) Strictly family
(c) Clinicians/staff only
(d) Only by the individual

___ 8. _____ denotes a set of behaviors that are genetically determined and are associated with a particular genetic disorder
(a) Diagnostic overshadowing
(b) Assessment procedure
(c) Behavioral phenotype
(d) Category

___ 9. A particular psychiatric disorder may be manifested differently between:
(a) Men and woman
(b) Different seasons
(c) Different levels of disability (mild/moderate vs. severe/profound)
(d) Different income levels

___ 10. Explanatory notes are based on
(a) Helping doctors keep track of patients
(b) Breaking down disorders for families to understand
(c) Separating care providers from staff
(d) Specific behavior characteristics in persons with IDD

Module VI

Support Strategies

Pre-Test

Chapter VI: Support Strategies

___ 1. People's inappropriate or challenging behaviors are _____; they meet a need or serve a purpose for them.
   (a) functional
   (b) permanent
   (c) evolving
   (d) opportunistic

___ 2. Choose the Components of a Positive Behavior Supports Approach:
   (a) Data collection, physical exam, punishers
   (b) Medication therapy, a behaviorist, positive praise
   (c) Comprehensive data, positive attention, an extinction plan
   (d) Functional assessment, comprehensive intervention, focus on quality of life and wellness

___ 3. Carlos loves going shopping for sneakers but he punches his staff when the store gets too crowded and he wants to leave the store. Considering PBS approaches, choose the best intervention for Carlos:
   (a) Do not allow Carlos to go shopping for sneakers any more
   (b) Pay attention to when the store becomes crowded and be proactive in leaving
   (c) Teach Carlos to ask to leave when he is ready
   (d) B and/or C

___ 4. Which of the following support strategies involves confirming the person's emotions?
   (a) Exploring
   (b) Validating
   (c) Active listening
   (d) All of the above

___ 5. Identify the rational approach to psychopharmacological treatment in individuals with ID/MI:
   (a) Medication can directly affect or stop or control maladaptive behavior
   (b) A psychiatric diagnosis isn't necessary for medication therapy as long as aggression is present
   (c) Treatment with medication is used to target the effects of a specific diagnosis
   (d) No other supports or accommodations are needed once a person is given the right medication

___ 6. Which of the following accurately describes the guiding principle of Self Determination?
   (a) When individuals with IDD have choice and control in their lives they experience increased community integration, as well as increases in adaptive behavior.
   (b) When individuals with IDD have choice and control in their lives they experience increased community integration, as well as increases in problem behavior.
   (c) When individuals with IDD have choice and control in their lives they experience decreased community integration, as well as increases in problem behavior.
   (d) When individuals with IDD have choice and control in their lives they experience increased community integration, as well as more stress and anxiety over choice making.

___ 7. The purpose of _____ is to help the individual self-manage tension and/or anger, and well as distract the person from the source of stress and focus on an appropriate behavior.
   (a) Validation
   (b) Relaxation
   (c) Medication
   (d) Choice

___ 8. An effective communication strategy to help deescalate in a positive way includes putting the choice back to the person. What does that entail?
   (a) Remind the person that he or she is engaging in an inappropriate behavior
   (b) Review for the person the potential consequences if the escalation continues
   (c) Remind the person of the more productive and effective choices that can be made
   (d) Ask the person to choose how long they are going to take to deescalate

___ 9. Medication complications, inadequate or inappropriate supports, and mental health symptoms are risk factors that contribute to:
   (a) Power struggles and aggression
   (b) People with Dual Diagnosis experiencing a crisis
   (c) Environmental triggers of problem behaviors
   (d) Improved quality of life

___ 10 A crisis plan should include:
   (a) A clear description of what constitutes the crisis for the person
   (b) Clearly outlines actions to be taken by whom at points along the path as crisis unfolds
   (c) Contact information for the resources and people to contact when a crisis occurs
   (d) All of the above

Slide 1

Module VI

Support Strategies

Slide 2

Support Strategies

In this module, we will discuss the following advanced support strategies:

1. Positive Behavior Supports
2. Communication Tone
3. Environmental
4. Choice and self determination
5. Relaxation techniques
6. Verbal strategies

Slide 3

Learning Objectives

- Discuss 5 principles for achieving a therapeutic relationship
- Name 3 special considerations when conducting therapy with people who have IDD/MI
- Describe 5 predictable crises
- Summarize 3 crisis management strategies
- Describe the main characteristics and components of Positive Behavior Supports
- Describe the importance of communication and setting tone when supporting a person with IDD
- List and describe verbal and non-verbal de-escalation support strategies

Slide 4

Positive Behavior Supports

Positive Behavior Support

(PBS) involves the changing situations and events that people with problem behaviors experience in order to reduce the likelihood of their occurrence and increase social, personal, and professional quality in their lives.

Slide 5

Positive Behavior Support

What does PBS Consider?

- Values about the rights and dignity of people who have disabilities and self-determination
- Practical science about how learning and behavior change occur
- Biomedical concerns
- Lifestyle concerns
- Changes in systems of support
- Team-based approaches

Slide 6

Positive Behavior Supports

Considerations (continued)

- Decrease negative behaviors
- Support appropriate behavior
- Focus on improving environment, not "fixing" people
- Quality of life enhancement
- Increase learning and independence
- Successful input and collaboration from those closest to the person and the person themselves
- Cooperation across disciplines

Slide 7

Positive Behavior Supports

Components of a PBS Approach

- Functional Assessment
- Comprehensive Intervention
- Focus on Quality of Life and Wellness

Slide 8

Support Strategies

1. The Importance of Communication:
   Setting the Tone
   - Begin your interaction socially.
   - **Use a non-demanding approach.**
   - Give choices whenever possible.

Slide 9

Support Strategies

2. Environmental Contributors to Problem Behaviors
   - Important to evaluate the environment
   - Look for things that might be contributing to, or triggering, problem behaviors

NOTE:

Important to look at environment from the person's perspective.

Slide 10

Support Strategies
Exercise

Activity: *Consider environmental contributors and solutions for the following behaviors*

• Eduardo has been removing his clothes in the classroom. This only occurs in the winter months when he is often wearing sweaters.

• Laura will scream and bite her hand at the kitchen table during meal times.

• Angel bangs his head against the window on the school bus. Recently, the bus changed routes so this changed the order of his pick up and the location of his seat on the bus.

Slide 11

Support Strategies

3. Providing Choice and Self Determination

Guiding Principle: Choice has positive benefits

- increases community integration
- increases adaptive behavior
- improves overall quality of life
- decreases problem behavior

Slide 12

Support Strategies

4. Relaxation Techniques

The purpose is to help the individual self manage and reduce stress, tension and/or angry feelings.

Relaxation strategies distract the person from the source of the stress and place focus on appropriate behavior.

Slide 13

Relaxation

Let's practice together
PMR: Progressive Muscle Relaxation

Sit in a relaxed position
Focus on yourself and on achieving relaxation in specific body muscles.
Tune out all other thoughts
Squeeze fists together tightly. Slowly count to five and release
Shrug your shoulders up to your ears for five seconds. Relax.
Arch your back off the floor for five seconds. Relax.
Squeeze legs tightly and slowly count to 5 and release
Repeat for other body parts that are tense
Avoid body parts that are sore of uncomfortable

Slide 14

What do you find relaxing?

Activity: Think of an activity that you find relaxing:
- Playing an instrument? Listening to music? Attending concert?
- Taking a walk or hiking?
- Word puzzles or board games?
- Dancing, aerobics, jogging or other exercise?
- Watching TV? Going to the movies?
- Cooking, reading, sewing, scrapbooking

Using your interest and familiarity, design an activity for an individual or group in the setting where you work that promotes proactive relaxation opportunities. Build the most successful ideas into your regular routine!

Slide 15

Support Strategies

5. Verbal Strategy
- Verbal techniques can help an individual feel acknowledged and supported

- Verbal techniques can be used by direct care staff as well as clinical staff
    a. Validating
    b. Exploring
    c. Problem Solving

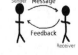

Slide 16

Support Strategies

5. a) Validating

Validating involves confirming the person's emotions.

An example of this is shown in the following scenario:

Jack: "Everybody around here hates me!"

Staff: "It sounds as though you are pretty angry."

Slide 17

Support Strategies

5. b) Validating & Exploring

Validating and Exploring can be combined and involve encouraging the individual to further explain whatever it is the individual is trying to communicate

An example of this is shown in the following scenario:

Jack: "Everybody around here hates me!"

Staff: "It sounds like you are pretty angry. Can you tell me what you are so mad about?"

Slide 18

Support Strategies

5. c) Problem Solving

- Identify the nature of the problem from the client's point of view.
- Explore alternative solutions to the problem
- Implement the best alternative solution

Slide 19

Support Strategies

Exercise: Verbal Strategies

You are working with a woman named Lorraine who believes that one of her staff or roommates steals her clothes from the laundry room. As a result she will no longer wash her clothes, wearing the same soiled outfits to work every day. When you approach Lorraine about this, she screams and yells about people stealing and not trusting anyone to help her.

Activity: consider the 3 verbal strategies reviewed on the prior slides to help Lorraine feel acknowledged and supported in reaching a productive and positive outcome.

Slide 20

Effective Communication Strategies

There are certain communication techniques which can be very helpful in de-escalating situations. These include:

1. Active Listening
2. Empathetic responses
3. Maintain a non-judgmental attitude

Slide 21

Effective Communication Strategies

4. Recognize and avoid power struggles

5. Watch your posture and body language

6. Validate feelings

7. Put the choices back to the person

Slide 22

Crisis Prevention and Planning

People who have a Dual Diagnosis are at risk of experiencing a crisis for a number of reasons:
- Medications/medical complications
- Changing life circumstances
- Inappropriate/inadequate supports
- Increase in mental health symptoms
- Substance abuse problems
- Behavioral phenotypes of genetic disorders

Slide 23

Crisis Prevention and Planning

By addressing environmental, biological, psychological and social factors that may contribute to problem behavior, staff may be able to assist the person to cope, maintain control of his/her own behavior, and learn positive, productive ways that address the function of the behavior.

Slide 24

Crisis Prevention and Planning

Ensure the plan includes a description of what a crisis is for a specific person

Outline the appropriate actions to address the issues at the earliest possible stage of the crisis unfolding.

The plan should also include appropriate intervention strategies that are effective when dealing with problem behavior.

Slide 25

Crisis Management

Non-Verbal De-Escalation Strategies

1. Monitor your body position and body language

2. Avoid physically putting yourself in harm's way

3. Maintain a demeanor of calmness, neutrality, and confidence

Slide 26

Crisis Management

Verbal De-Escalation Strategies

1. Use a calm tone of voice

2. Use reflective listening

3. Avoid threatening punishment

4. Avoid power struggles

5. Do not ignore escalations of behaviors that could lead to severe behaviors

Continued . . .

Slide 27

Crisis Management

Verbal De-Escalation Strategies

6. Change staffing if necessary

7. Affirm that you understand

8. Change the subject if it appears to agitate the person more to talk about it (i.e., offer a drink of water, bring up an topic that interests him or her such as sporting event or TV program)

Slide 28

Crisis Management
Verbal De-Escalation Strategies

9. Change aspects of the environment.

10. Set limits by reminding the person of the choices and outcomes but do so in a firm, fair manner and with a non-emotional tone of voice.

11. Remind the individual of the desirable consequences of choosing a positive behavior as opposed to a problem behavior. Then remind the persons of the undesirable consequences that can occur if he or she engages in the problem behavior.

McGivery & Sweetland, 2011

Slide 29

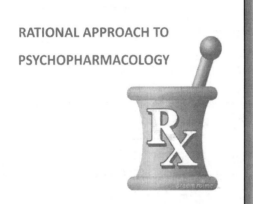

RATIONAL APPROACH TO PSYCHOPHARMACOLOGY

Slide 30

MYTH: MEDICATION TREATMENT IS USED TO CONTROL MALADAPTIVE BEHAVIORS

<u>Premise:</u>
Medication-based therapies directly affect behavior.

<u>Reality:</u>
Behaviors such as self-injury and aggression are too nonspecific to be considered as direct targets for drug therapy.

<u>Treatment implications:</u>
The appropriate targets for medication therapy are the changes in neurophysiological function that mediate behavior associated with psychiatric disorders.

Slide 31

Medication Treatment

Pharmacotherapy is therapeutic and may be the first choice treatment for some psychiatric disorders:

- Major depression
- Mania states
- Schizophrenia

Medication treatment should be diagnostically related to a DSM 5 diagnostic and treatment guideline or the DM-ID.

Slide 32

Putting it all together

Activity: Develop a blueprint wellness plan for someone you support. Consider the support strategies reviewed in this chapter that would apply to him/her.

Tips
- Identity the person's strengths and interests
- Consider the person's diagnosis and mental health needs
- Promote relaxation opportunities
- Anticipate challenges and be prepared with de-escalation and validation strategies
- Build in ways to help the person feel good about him/herself and develop positive identify
- Monitor behavior and medication information

MODULE VI

Post-Test

Chapter VI: Support Strategies

___ 1. People's inappropriate or challenging behaviors are _____; they meet a need or serve a purpose for them.
    (a) functional
    (b) permanent
    (c) evolving
    (d) opportunistic

___ 2. Choose the Components of a Positive Behavior Supports Approach:
    (a) Data collection, physical exam, punishers
    (b) Medication therapy, a behaviorist, positive praise
    (c) Comprehensive data, positive attention, an extinction plan
    (d) Functional assessment, comprehensive intervention, focus on quality of life and wellness

___ 3. Carlos loves going shopping for sneakers but he punches his staff when the store gets too crowded and he wants to leave the store. Considering PBS approaches, choose the best intervention for Carlos:
    (a) Do not allow Carlos to go shopping for sneakers any more
    (b) Pay attention to when the store becomes crowded and be proactive in leaving
    (c) Teach Carlos to ask to leave when he is ready
    (d) B and/or C

___ 4. Which of the following support strategies involves confirming the person's emotions?
    (a) Exploring
    (b) Validating
    (c) Active listening
    (d) All of the above

___ 5. Identify the rational approach to psychopharmacological treatment in individuals with ID/MI:
    (a) Medication can directly affect or stop or control maladaptive behavior
    (b) A psychiatric diagnosis isn't necessary for medication therapy as long as aggression is present
    (c) Treatment with medication is used to target the effects of a specific diagnosis
    (d) No other supports or accommodations are needed once a person is given the right medication

___ 6. Which of the following accurately describes the guiding principle of Self Determination?
   (a) When individuals with IDD have choice and control in their lives they experience increased community integration, as well as increases in adaptive behavior.
   (b) When individuals with IDD have choice and control in their lives they experience increased community integration, as well as increases in problem behavior.
   (c) When individuals with IDD have choice and control in their lives they experience decreased community integration, as well as increases in problem behavior.
   (d) When individuals with IDD have choice and control in their lives they experience increased community integration, as well as more stress and anxiety over choice making.

___ 7. The purpose of _____ is to help the individual self-manage tension and/or anger, and well as distract the person from the source of stress and focus on an appropriate behavior.
   (a) Validation
   (b) Relaxation
   (c) Medication
   (d) Choice

___ 8. An effective communication strategy to help deescalate in a positive way includes putting the choice back to the person. What does that entail?
   (a) Remind the person that he or she is engaging in an inappropriate behavior
   (b) Review for the person the potential consequences if the escalation continues
   (c) Remind the person of the more productive and effective choices that can be made
   (d) Ask the person to choose how long they are going to take to deescalate

___ 9. Medication complications, inadequate or inappropriate supports, and mental health symptoms are risk factors that contribute to:
   (a) Power struggles and aggression
   (b) People with Dual Diagnosis experiencing a crisis
   (c) Environmental triggers of problem behaviors
   (d) Improved quality of life

___ 10 A crisis plan should include:
   (a) A clear description of what constitutes the crisis for the person
   (b) Clearly outlines actions to be taken by whom at points along the path as crisis unfolds
   (c) Contact information for the resources and people to contact when a crisis occurs
   (d) All of the above

Module VII

Adapting Therapy for People with IDD

Pre-Test

Module VII – Adapted Therapies Pre/Post Test

___ 1. When adapting therapy for a person with IDD/MI, which of the following statements is true.
   (a) The therapist needs to take safety precautions for therapy sessions because a client with IDD/MI will become aggressive.
   (b) The therapist should determine what makes a particular intellectual activity difficult for the person and develop an appropriate adaptation of that activity or use as alternate activity.
   (c) The therapist does not need to address any historical abuse or trauma because people with IDD do not experience hurt or trauma from exploitation or abuse like non-disabled people do.
   (d) The therapist should treat the person with IDD as if they were a child and always use language and techniques used with children.

___ 2. Complete the sentence with the most appropriate response. A person with IDD may seek therapy _____
   (a) For reasons as varied as the reasons for which people without an IDD seek therapy.
   (b) For minor issues. People with IDD do not have the same types of problems that are experienced by people without and IDD.
   (c) When their support staff have thoroughly assessed and diagnosed their maladaptive behavior on the internet.
   (d) When they have the memory retention and self-awareness to participate in traditional, non-adapted models of therapy.

___ 3. Which of the following is false? Whether or not trauma leads to longer term issues and lasting stress can depend on
   (a) The intensity of the stressor
   (b) A person's inherent resilience or vulnerability
   (c) The gender of the person who experienced the trauma
   (d) The time of day the trauma occurred.

___ 4. Complete the sentence with the most appropriate response. Experiences that can lead to longer term trauma for a person with IDD _____
   (a) Can be related to the buildup of every day stresses and losses that can be unique to their experience.
   (b) Occur infrequently because people with IDD do not have the ability to experience most situations as traumatic.
   (c) Are not as frequent as they are for the general population due to the limited life experiences of a person with IDD.
   (d) None of the responses are appropriate to complete the sentence.

___ 5. Identify the false statement below.
   (a) CBT (Cognitive Behavior Therapy) has yielded positive results amongst people with IDD.
   (b) The general under-diagnosis of PTSD amongst people who have an IDD leads to a large portion of those with PTSD never receiving treatment.
   (c) Positive identity development can be an effective trauma informed intervention.
   (d) EMDR is not a recommended treatment for people with IDD who have experienced trauma.

___ 6. Which of the following statements about Positive Identity Development is false?
   (a) Positive Identity Development refers to one's sense of self that develops through the accumulation of experience, the integration of experiences, and interpretation of experiences.
   (b) Many people with an IDD have a largely negative sense of identity, which is constituted of all the good things the person is not.
   (c) For a person with IDD, EMDR can be effective in supporting the person to develop a positive sense of self, which can reduce the risk of the person experiencing a traumatic event.
   (d) All of the above statements are false.

___ 7. Using DBT (Dialectical Behavior Therapy) for trauma treatment, focuses on
   (a) Mindfulness, emotional regulation, distress tolerance, and interpersonal effectiveness.
   (b) Integration of both psychological and psychotherapies into a standard set of procedures and clinical protocols.
   (c) Supported positive identity development, mindfulness, distress tolerance and interpersonal effectiveness.
   (d) Skill development and more adaptive cognitive appraisals of events that trigger intense response with strategies presented in a variety of concrete media.

___ 8. CBT (Cognitive Behavior Therapy) is effective in helping improve a person's overall functioning through
   (a) Mindfulness practice
   (b) Engaging subconscious processes and use of archetypal therapy
   (c) Applied Behavior Analytic interventions
   (d) Skill development and more adaptive cognitive appraisals of events that trigger intense response with strategies presented in a variety of concrete media.

___ 9. Individual Psychotherapy is most effective for people with IDD when the clinician
   (a) Focuses on increasing distress tolerance through a standard set of procedures and clinical protocols.
   (b) Adapts a standard technique to the client's cognitive level and engage significant others in the therapeutic process.
   (c) Focuses on skill development and more adaptive cognitive appraisals of events that trigger intense response with strategies presented in a variety of concrete media.
   (d) None of the above

___ 10. Finish the sentence with the most appropriate response. Group therapy for people with IDD who have experienced trauma _____
   (a) Helps people foster meaningful relationships, establish a sense of trust, and helps decrease feelings of inadequacy and loneliness.
   (b) Is not beneficial, as people with IDD cannot benefit from insight-oriented group therapy.
   (c) Adapts a standard, uniform technique and engages significant others in the therapeutic process.
   (d) All of the above

MENTAL HEALTH APPROACHES TO INTELLECTUAL/DEVELOPMENTAL DISABILITY:

MODULE VII

Slide 1

Module VII

Adapting Therapy for People with IDD

Slide 2

This module introduces concepts in Adapting Therapy to make it more useful for persons with IDD.

This modules discusses concepts in mental wellness.

Slide 3

Learning Objectives

- List reasons why people with IDD seek therapy
- List ways to make therapy more accessible to people with IDD
- Describe the principles and benefits of DBT, CBT and Individual /Group Therapy
- Describe how trauma effects people with IDD
- Describe the trauma treatment strategies and adaptations for IDD
- Describe how to support a person in positive Identity Development

Slide 4

Adapted Therapies

Myth: Persons with IDD are not appropriate for psychotherapy

Premise: Impairments in cognitive abilities and language skills make psychotherapy ineffective.

Reality: Level of intelligence is not a sole indicator for appropriateness of therapy.

Treatment Applications: Psychotherapy approaches need to be adapted to the expressive and receptive language skills of the person.

Slide 5

Adapted Therapies

- Relationship between a client and a therapist/counselor

- **Engaged in a therapeutic relationship**

- To achieve a change in emotions, thoughts or behavior

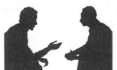

Slide 6

Similarities Between Children without IDD And Adults with IDD

Without IDD	With IDD
6-7 Years Old	6-7 Years Old Cognitive Level Mild IDD Borderline IDD

Both usually dependent on others

Both tend to be in supervised settings

Both have cognitive limitations in terms of:
- Problem solving
- Impulse control
- Concrete thought

Slide 7

Similarities Between Children without IDD And Adults with IDD

- Both struggle with issues of:
    - Independence
    - Peer group
    - Identity choices
    - Vocational
    - Sexual identity
    - Authority issues

- Both referred to therapy by others

Slide 8

Why People with and without IDD Seek Therapy

Interpersonal Concerns	22%
General Psychological Functioning	18%
Work	12%
Sexuality	6%
Family	5%
Residential Living & Adjustment	5%
Behavior	4%
Financial & Material Resources	4%
Accepting & Coping with Disability	4%
Dealing with Authority Figures	4%
Other	16%

Slide 9

Adapted Therapies

Cognitive Load of Therapy and Intervention

Cognitive Load refers to the amount of information and interactions processed simultaneously (or) thinking and reasoning required for people to build on what they already understand.

- Many of the typical ways we provide therapy are complex and require significant cognitive functioning to work
- Typical practices may not work for a person with IDD.

Slide 10

Adapted Therapies

Many typical therapy sessions start with this question: "Have you been feeling better since last time I saw you?"

- Must remember feelings from last visit
- Must know current feelings
- Must be able to compare
- Must know what the therapist is really asking
- Must be able to inductively reason

And so on and so on…

Slide 11

Adapted Therapies

Therapy Can Be Made Accessible

- Accessibility doesn't just refer to physical access
- The term applies just as easily to intellectual and cognitive access
- Special educators do this on a daily basis. From their practices we find:
- "Go slow, be concrete, repeat" is a recommendation that is often applied to counseling and therapy with persons with an intellectual disability (Morasky, 2007).

Slide 12

Therapeutic Principles

- Empathetic understanding
- Respect and acceptance of client
- Concreteness
- Be consistent
- Confidentiality
- Draw the client out
- Express genuine interest in your client
- Be aware of your own feelings

Slide 13

Confidentiality

- Nothing discussed in therapy will be released without the person's permission

- With the client's permission, the therapist will work collaboratively other care providers

Slide 14

Adapted Therapy

Adaptations

Intellectual activities that often pose challenges for people who have dual diagnosis:
- speed,
- number,
- complexity,
- abstraction,
- reasoning
- generalization
- decision making

WARNING CHALLENGES AHEAD

Slide 15

Therapy Model

Help People Better Cope With Problems

1. Listen
2. Reflect
3. Probe
4. Support
5. Facilitate problem solving
6. Evaluate outcome

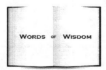

Slide 16

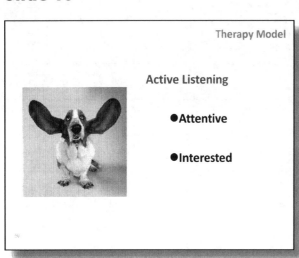

Therapy Model

Active Listening

- Attentive
- Interested

Slide 17

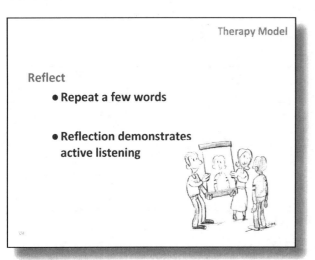

Therapy Model

Reflect
- Repeat a few words
- Reflection demonstrates active listening

Slide 18

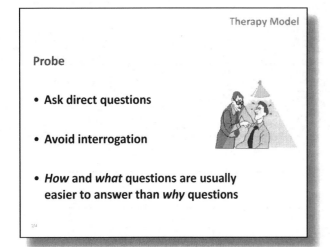

Therapy Model

Probe
- Ask direct questions
- Avoid interrogation
- *How* and *what* questions are usually easier to answer than *why* questions

Slide 19

Therapy Model

Support

- Supportive statements indicate understanding
- Express that you care
- Acknowledge having been in a similar situation

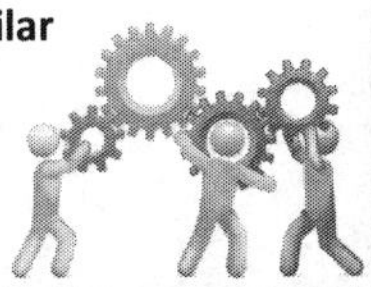

Slide 20

Exercise

Pair up and practice active listening. Each person gets to be the speaker and the listener. Make sure to use all of the active listening strategies described on the previous slides.

Slide 21

Therapy Model

Facilitate problem solving

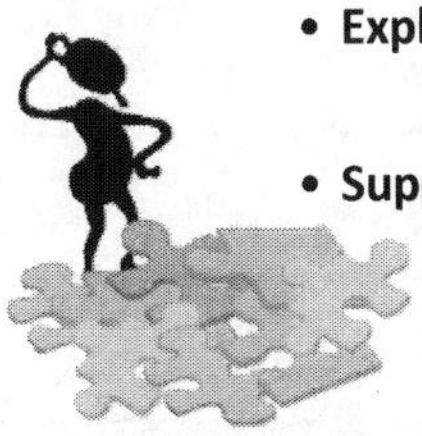

- Explore alternative options
- Support acceptable solutions

Slide 22

Therapy Model

Evaluate outcome
- Was outcome acceptable?
- Was it positive?
- What was learned?

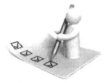

Slide 23

Best Practice

Best Practice in Adapting Therapy for people who have an IDD.

1. Person-centered thinking (Illness Management and Recovery?)
a. Work with individual to identify specific support needs
b. Arrange support to address those
c. Individual supports

Slide 24

Best Practice

...Continued

2. Wellness approaches
a. Support organized into wellness promotion
b. Assist with healthy lifestyle and activity

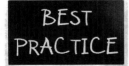

Slide 25

Best Practice

...Continued

3. Positive behavior supports

a. Management of problem behavior relies upon identifying reasons for problem behavior

b. Look into different areas of life in terms of understanding problem behaviors

c. Intervention targets strength based planning, support

d. Identification, teaching and wellness approaches

Slide 26

Best Practice

4. Adapting Instruction in General

- Size
- Time
- Level of Support
- Input
- Difficulty
- Output
- Participation
- Alternate
- Substitute Curriculum

Slide 27

Adaptations

Size

Adapt the number of items that the person is expected to learn or complete.

General example: If person is to know the fifty states, have persons only be responsible for remembering a certain number at a time. This would be dependent on the person's level of disability.

Therapeutic Example: In doing the "Three Good Things" intervention from Positive Psychology, the client is asked to only generate "One Good Thing."

Slide 28

Adaptations

Time
Adapt the time allotted and allowed for learning, task completion, or testing.

For example: Allow person additional time to complete timed assignments. However, if the total project is due by a particular time, have the person complete each portion of the project over various intervals with the required finished project due at a later time.

Therapeutic Example: The client is allowed extra time to answer questions.

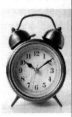

Deschenes, Ebeling, & Sprague, 1994

Slide 29

Adaptations

Level of Support
Increase the amount of personal assistance with a specific person.

For example: Allow for peer teaching. Pair the slower persons with the more advanced persons in order to provide support.

Therapeutic Example: In Narrative Therapy, the client is given additional prompting and reminders.

Deschenes, Ebeling, & Sprague, 1994

Slide 30

Adaptations

Input
Adapt the way instruction is delivered to the person.

For example: Provide persons with a audio and/or video tape of the lesson. Allow for field trips, guest speakers, peer teaching, computer support, video productions.

Therapeutic Example: Concrete objects can be used in Cognitive Behavior Therapy.

Deschenes, Ebeling, & Sprague, 1994

Slide 31

Difficulty — Adaptations
Reduce the difficult of the Task

For example: Allow the person to be creative providing that task is completed according to instructor's specifications. For example the person may draw a picture of the assignment, do an interview, etc. depending on subject. Allow the person to come up with the idea. Accept any reasonable modifications.

Therapeutic Example: Allow the person to use a variety of different relaxation responses.

Slide 32

Output — Adaptations
Adapt how the person can respond to instruction.

For example: Allow persons to draw pictures, write an essay, complete specific computer software program relating to lesson.

Therapeutic Example: Allow the client to draw responses or use a communication device to answer questions. A menu board of responses offers a choice of answers, reducing the need for crude recall.

Slide 33

Participation — Adaptations
Adapt the extent to which a person is actively involved in the task.

For example: Tailor the person's participation in a task to his or her abilities, whether intellectual or physical.

Therapeutic Example: Adapt Wellness Interventions, such as the promotion of experienced creativity, to include Partial Participation.

Slide 34

Adaptations

Alternate

Adapt the goals or outcome expectations while using the same materials.

For example: In a writing assignment, alter the expectations for a disabled person who takes longer to write a paragraph.

Therapeutic Example: Allow them to dictate a Gratitude Letter as opposed to writing it themselves.

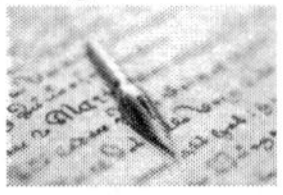

Slide 35

Adaptations

Substitute Curriculum

Provide different instruction and materials to meet a person's individual goals.

For example: Instead of discussing the reasons for the civil war, have the disabled person work on a puzzle showing the Union and Confederate states.

Therapeutic Example: Teach coping instruction using simpler, less abstract example.

Slide 36

Exercise

Get in small groups of 3-4. If you were going to teach a person with IDD to make a paper airplane, consider how to use each of the different adaptations from slide 26 to simplify the instruction.

Slide 37

Psychological Interventions

Recommendations Specific for Therapy for Persons with IDD

- Morasky (2007) has provided an excellent description of strategies for adapting psychological intervention for persons with IDD, including modifying speed, number, abstraction, and complexity.

    – Morasky, R. (2007). Making counseling/therapy intellectually attainable. *The NADD Bulletin*, *10*, pp. 58-62.

Slide 38

Psychological Interventions

Guiding Principles:

- Use language that promotes hope
- Raise expectations of what people are capable of accomplishing
- Stay focused on strengths

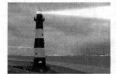

Slide 39

Psychological Interventions

- Build everyone's hope
- Instill a source of hope whenever possible
- Feeling a sense of hope for the future can be transformative

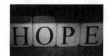

Slide 40

Psychological Interventions

- Celebrate accomplishments

- Find ways to listen to our consumers

Slide 41

Trauma Informed Intervention

Trauma
- Trauma is the emotional response to a terrible event like an accident, rape or natural disaster.
- Immediately after the event, shock and denial are typical.
- Longer term reactions include unpredictable emotions, flashbacks, strained relationships and even physical symptoms like headaches or nausea (APA, 2013).

Slide 42

Trauma Informed Intervention

A major trauma could be
- Sexual Assault/Physical Assault
- Natural or manmade disasters
- Catastrophic illness
- Loss of a loved one
- Humiliation
- Bullying
- Deprivation and powerlessness to act on one's own behalf

Slide 43

Trauma Informed Intervention

Trauma

People with intellectual/developmental disabilities are at greater risk for being victimized or abused.

Some experts believe as many as 90% of people with intellectual disabilities have some level of traumatic stress. Sobsey (1994) reports that people with disabilities are twice as likely to experience abuse.

Slide 44

Trauma Informed Intervention

People with IDD often manifest PTSD differently than what is typically recognized as PTSD in the DSM – V

Some individuals may have flashbacks, but are not able to communicate that experience. What they do communicate, rather, may be misunderstood as a psychotic disorder.

Slide 45

Trauma Informed Intervention

Simple and Complex PTSD

Big T traumas:
 simple post-traumatic stress resulting from a one-time incident — such as a rape, violent assault, injury

Little t Traumas:
 complex post-traumatic stress is a complex set of responses that follows chronic, multiple, and/or ongoing traumatic events such as taunting, teasing, tormenting, prolonged abuse

Slide 46

Trauma Informed Intervention

Trauma Informed Intervention
- Positive Identity Development
- DBT – Dialectical Behavior Therapy
  - Supportive Counseling
  - Group Therapy
- TF-CBT
- EMDR
- Individual Psychotherapy

Slide 47

Positive Identity Development

Positive Identity Development

The presence of an intellectual/developmental disability impacts exposure to new experiences and the person's understanding and integration of those experiences.

This requires the organization and delivery of identity-related supports and counseling for persons with IDD across the lifespan.

Harvey, 2000

ISlide 48

Positive Identity Development

Many people with an IDD have a largely negative sense of identity which is constituted of all the good things the person is not. Specific therapeutic approaches can help to create a more positive sense of identity.

Harvey, 2008

Slide 49

Positive Identity Development

"The therapist facilitates the discovery of self and then helps to strengthen and reinforce that sense of self from session to session."

Karen Harvey, 2009

Slide 50

EMDR

Eye Movement Desensitization and Reprocessing (EMDR)

First developed by Francine Shapiro upon noticing that certain eye movements reduced the intensity of disturbing thought.

EMDR uses a person's own rapid, rhythmic eye movements.

Treatment consists of 8 phases with precise intentions.

Slide 51

Dialectical Behavior Therapy

Dialectical Behavior Therapy (DBT)

DBT is a comprehensive treatment program addressing deficits in emotion regulation, distress tolerance, and interpersonal relationships accomplished through:
- individual psychotherapy,
- skills training groups, and
- supervision/case consultation groups

Slide 52

Dialectical Behavior Therapy

Using DBT, therapists have five main tasks:

- expand client capabilities,
- motivate the client to engage in new behaviors,
- generalize the use of the new behaviors,
- establish a treatment environment that reinforces progress, and
- maintain capable and motivated therapists

Slide 53

Therapeutic Effects Of Group Therapy

13 Benefits

1. Fosters meaningful relationships
2. Increases relationship skills
3. Promotes problem solving skills
4. Enables learning through observation

Slide 54

Therapeutic Effects Of Group Therapy
13 Benefits

5. Helps decrease feelings of: inadequacy, isolation and defeat
6. Promotes peer support
7. Fosters a sense of security
8. Promotes group cohesiveness
9. Establishes sense of trust

Slide 55

Therapeutic Effects Of Group Therapy

13 Benefits

10. Promotes sense of belonging – shared experiences

11. Instills sense of hope - optimism

12. Facilitates altruism – helping others

13. Promotes self understanding

Slide 56

Cognitive Behavior Therapy

Cognitive Behavioral Therapy (CBT)

CBT is effective in helping clients improve functioning and in identifying the beliefs, feelings, and behaviors associated with the trauma responses.

Overall functioning is improved through skills development and more adaptive cognitive appraisals of events that trigger intense responses.

CBT teaches people to monitor thoughts and change thought patterns leading to problems. There is a strong evidence base showing utility for persons with IDD if proper adaptation is made (Gaus, 2007).

Slide 57

Individual Psychotherapy

Individual Psychotherapy

Individual psychotherapy aims to increase the person's overall well being.

It is most effective when the therapist adapts the model to consider the cognitive ability of the person with intellectual/developmental disability.

Slide 58

Adapted Therapies

When implementing adapted therapies with people who have IDD, remember to:
- Slow down your speech
- Use language that is comprehensible to the person
- Present information one item at a time using different methods (visual, auditory)
- Take frequent pauses during the session to check comprehension
- Use multisensory input

Continued....

Slide 59

Adapted Therapies

Continued....
- Make specific suggestions for change
- Allow time to practice new skills
- Use more repetition
- Do not assume that information will generalize to new situations and spend more time working on generalization
- Do not assume the information is too complex for the person to understand

Slide 60

Adapted Therapy

"Contracting"

Contracting is an informal counseling tool which outlines the understanding of both the client and the therapist about the process and expectations. It basically means, "We are on the same page about how this is going to go."

Considerations for inclusion in the contract:
- Ask for permission to interrupt,
- Avoid using inappropriate language
- Types of tips people who have IDD will find useful regarding the therapy process.

Slide 61

By adapting empirically validated psychotherapy techniques and treatments, a clinician can provide effective therapy for people with an IDD and MI.

With some consideration to cognitive abilities, including expressive and receptive language, psychotherapy techniques can be effectively adapted to meet the needs of people who have an IDD and an MI.

MODULE VII

Post-Test

Module VII – Adapted Therapies Pre/Post Test

___ 1. When adapting therapy for a person with IDD/MI, which of the following statements is true.
   (a) The therapist needs to take safety precautions for therapy sessions because a client with IDD/MI will become aggressive.
   (b) The therapist should determine what makes a particular intellectual activity difficult for the person and develop an appropriate adaptation of that activity or use as alternate activity.
   (c) The therapist does not need to address any historical abuse or trauma because people with IDD do not experience hurt or trauma from exploitation or abuse like non-disabled people do.
   (d) The therapist should treat the person with IDD as if they were a child and always use language and techniques used with children.

___ 2. Complete the sentence with the most appropriate response. A person with IDD may seek therapy _____
   (a) For reasons as varied as the reasons for which people without an IDD seek therapy.
   (b) For minor issues. People with IDD do not have the same types of problems that are experienced by people without and IDD.
   (c) When their support staff have thoroughly assessed and diagnosed their maladaptive behavior on the internet.
   (d) When they have the memory retention and self-awareness to participate in traditional, non-adapted models of therapy.

___ 3. Which of the following is false? Whether or not trauma leads to longer term issues and lasting stress can depend on
   (a) The intensity of the stressor
   (b) A person's inherent resilience or vulnerability
   (c) The gender of the person who experienced the trauma
   (d) The time of day the trauma occurred.

___ 4. Complete the sentence with the most appropriate response. Experiences that can lead to longer term trauma for a person with IDD _____
   (a) Can be related to the buildup of every day stresses and losses that can be unique to their experience.
   (b) Occur infrequently because people with IDD do not have the ability to experience most situations as traumatic.
   (c) Are not as frequent as they are for the general population due to the limited life experiences of a person with IDD.
   (d) None of the responses are appropriate to complete the sentence.

___ 5. Identify the false statement below.
   (a) CBT (Cognitive Behavior Therapy) has yielded positive results amongst people with IDD.
   (b) The general under-diagnosis of PTSD amongst people who have an IDD leads to a large portion of those with PTSD never receiving treatment.
   (c) Positive identity development can be an effective trauma informed intervention.
   (d) EMDR is not a recommended treatment for people with IDD who have experienced trauma.

___ 6. Which of the following statements about Positive Identity Development is false?
   (a) Positive Identity Development refers to one's sense of self that develops through the accumulation of experience, the integration of experiences, and interpretation of experiences.
   (b) Many people with an IDD have a largely negative sense of identity, which is constituted of all the good things the person is not.
   (c) For a person with IDD, EMDR can be effective in supporting the person to develop a positive sense of self, which can reduce the risk of the person experiencing a traumatic event.
   (d) All of the above statements are false.

___ 7. Using DBT (Dialectical Behavior Therapy) for trauma treatment, focuses on
   (a) Mindfulness, emotional regulation, distress tolerance, and interpersonal effectiveness.
   (b) Integration of both psychological and psychotherapies into a standard set of procedures and clinical protocols.
   (c) Supported positive identity development, mindfulness, distress tolerance and interpersonal effectiveness.
   (d) Skill development and more adaptive cognitive appraisals of events that trigger intense response with strategies presented in a variety of concrete media.

___ 8. CBT (Cognitive Behavior Therapy) is effective in helping improve a person's overall functioning through
   (a) Mindfulness practice
   (b) Engaging subconscious processes and use of archetypal therapy
   (c) Applied Behavior Analytic interventions
   (d) Skill development and more adaptive cognitive appraisals of events that trigger intense response with strategies presented in a variety of concrete media.

___ 9. Individual Psychotherapy is most effective for people with IDD when the clinician
   (a) Focuses on increasing distress tolerance through a standard set of procedures and clinical protocols.
   (b) Adapts a standard technique to the client's cognitive level and engage significant others in the therapeutic process.
   (c) Focuses on skill development and more adaptive cognitive appraisals of events that trigger intense response with strategies presented in a variety of concrete media.
   (d) None of the above

___ 10. Finish the sentence with the most appropriate response. Group therapy for people with IDD who have experienced trauma _____
   (a) Helps people foster meaningful relationships, establish a sense of trust, and helps decrease feelings of inadequacy and loneliness.
   (b) Is not beneficial, as people with IDD cannot benefit from insight-oriented group therapy.
   (c) Adapts a standard, uniform technique and engages significant others in the therapeutic process.
   (d) All of the above

MODULE VII

Module VIII

Childhood and Adolescence

Pre-Test

Module VIII: Childhood and Adolescence

___ 1. Which of the following diagnostic sign is NOT a potential sign of a developmental delay in a newborn infant according to the American Academy of Pediatrics?
(a) Reaching for an object
(b) Lack of response to loud sounds
(c) No smile response
(d) Feeding difficulties

___ 2. Which of the following is a purpose of having recognized developmental milestones?
(a) To set instructional expectations for children
(b) They are a widely used diagnostic tool
(c) To give a general idea of the changes to expect as a child gets older
(d) They have no purpose

___ 3. What is the typical age of a toddler?
(a) 0 – 1 year
(b) 1 – 3 years
(c) 2 – 5 years
(d) 2 – 7 years

___ 4. Typical children learn how to manage wanting everything immediately. The developmental activity associated with this is:
(a) Attachment to Caregivers
(b) Developing sense of identity
(c) Developing empathy
(d) Delaying gratification

___ 5. Why is sexuality education important for youth with IDD?
(a) All sexual thought is inherently risky
(b) Youth with IDD are sexual beings
(c) They must be protected from all sexual activity
(d) It is not important

___ 6. Children with IDD are:
(a) More likely to be bullied than typical youth
(b) Never bullied because they are always monitored by adults
(c) Rarely bullied because society doesn't accept it
(d) Easily taught to stop bullying by teaching martial arts

___ 7. Which of the following is NOT a step in conflict resolution?
   (a) Gathering perspectives
   (b) Threatening violence
   (c) Gathering options
   (d) Creating an agreement

___ 8. Which of the following is a type of healthy risk taking?
   (a) Drug use
   (b) Self-mutilation
   (c) Smoking
   (d) None are

___ 9. Difficulties with self-esteem may include?
   (a) Body image
   (b) Shyness
   (c) Embarrassment
   (d) All of the above

___ 10. Which of the following is a central question in the development of identity?
   (a) Who am I?
   (b) What am I to do in life?
   (c) Both of these questions
   (d) Neither of those questions

Slide 1

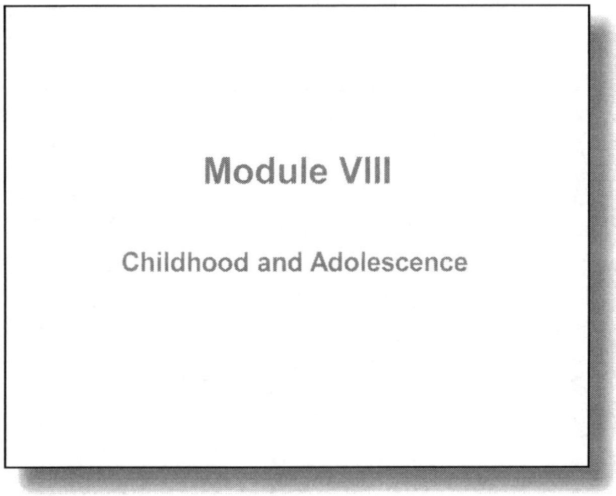

Module VIII

Childhood and Adolescence

Slide 2

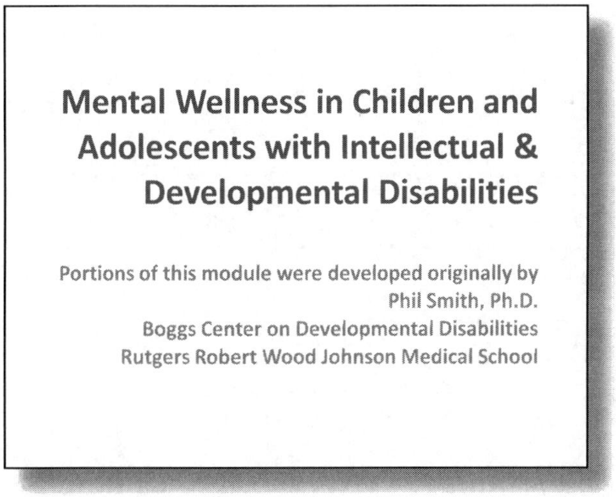

Mental Wellness in Children and Adolescents with Intellectual & Developmental Disabilities

Portions of this module were developed originally by
Phil Smith, Ph.D.
Boggs Center on Developmental Disabilities
Rutgers Robert Wood Johnson Medical School

Slide 3

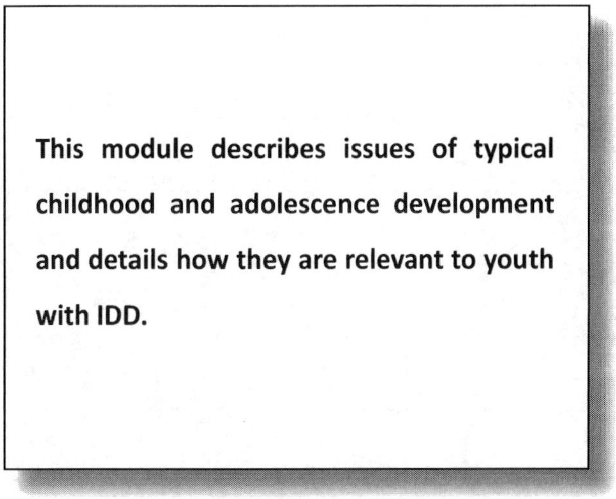

This module describes issues of typical childhood and adolescence development and details how they are relevant to youth with IDD.

Slide 4

Learning Objectives

- Describe issues around development for persons with IDD
- Describe the stages of typical development for younger children and adolescents
- Describe how disability effects self-image/self-esteem
- Describe the key milestones in sexuality and gender identity development
- Describe the impact of and support around various challenges of maturation

Slide 5

Childhood and Adolescence

Issues of Development

- There is a typical pathway or sequence of development in which certain cognitive, social, and emotional things are seen in each stage for typical people.
- Functioning and behavior are influenced by stages of development.
- Intellectual/developmental disabilities often change development due to difficulties in learning, different patterns of interaction, and lack of typical experiences, but most stages still occur (American Academy of Pediatrics, 2013b).

Slide 6

Childhood and Adolescence

Typical Stages

Approximate ages
- Newborn (ages 0–1 month)
- Infant (ages 1 month – 1 year)
- Toddler (ages 1–3 years)
- Preschooler (ages 4–6 years)
- School-aged child (ages 6–13 years)
- Adolescent (ages 13–20)

Slide 7

Characteristics of Typical Younger Children

- Often significant issues with attachment and attachment disorders
- Typical developmental tasks related to delaying gratification, task completion, and development of a sense of identify
- Many problems related to impulsiveness and lack of empathy

Slide 8

Characteristics of Adolescence

Teen life is complex for all young people
- Physically mature
- Sexually mature
- Emotionally mature
    - Desire independence
    - Sense of identity is built
    - Heightened focus on peers
    - Sexual awareness

Slide 9

Adolescence and Disability

An adolescent with an IDD experiences the same life complexities as other adolescents.

The presence of an IDD or physical disability can make learning and making sense of the world more complex.

Slide 10

Childhood and Adolescence
Self-image, Self-esteem

- Central theme – discovering oneself
  - Creating a personality
  - Shaping a personal image of oneself (very self-conscious)
  - Concerned with outward appearance

- Often focus on the ways they fail to meet the ideal
  - This often results in low self-esteem and unhappiness

- Shapes how they feel that peers look at them
- Use what one's peers think to determine their self-image
- Try out roles and test these out through social interaction

Slide 11

Childhood and Adolescence
Problems with Self-esteem

Often include:
- Body image
- Weight problems
- Shyness
- Embarrassment

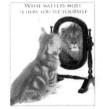

And for somebody with IDD, awareness of disability.

Slide 12

Exercise

Please come up with 10 words that describe you; 10 things that make you who you are.

Slide 13

Risk-taking Behavior
- All teenagers take risks as a normal part of growing up.
- Changes in the teen brain make risk-taking more likely
  - Time of great opportunity
  - Risks and problems as well
- Taking risks is a tool teens use to define and develop their identity
- Adolescents need to take risks
  - Healthy risk-taking can help prevent unhealthy risk-taking
  - Help create opportunities for healthy risks

Slide 14

Negative Risk-taking
- Drinking
- Smoking
- Unsafe sex
- Drug use
- Disordered eating
- Stealing
- Gang activity
- Self-mutilation

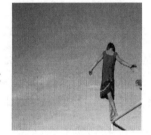

Slide 15

Healthy Risk-taking
- Sports
- Developing artistic abilities
- Volunteer activities
- Travel
- Making new friends
- Hobbies
- Exploring community

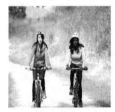

Slide 16

Exercise

- Identify 2 things you do that are examples of healthy risk taking.

- Then think of one negative risk-taking thing you do, but don't write it down or share it.

Slide 17

Childhood and Adolescence

Supporting Risk Taking

All such activities contain the possibility of failure.
- How can we help provide supports that include realistic goals?
- What skills do young people need to make good choices about taking risks?
- What are some challenges unique to younger individuals?

Slide 18

Childhood and Adolescence

Sexuality

- Key milestones of adolescent development
  - Attaining an adult body
    - Capable of reproducing
    - Intimate relationships
    - Complex emotions
- Individuals with disabilities may be hindered in this area of development
  - Functional limitations
  - Social isolation
    - Fewer social activities
    - Less likely to have intimate relationships
  - Lack of information on parenthood, birth control, and STDs

Slide 19

Development of Sexuality

- Children and adolescents with IDD, like all individuals, are sexual persons
- Most of their behaviors are "typical"
- The problem – often unable to distinguish between behaviors that are publicly and privately appropriate
- Attention to medical, functional, and behavioral issues may shift focus away from addressing sexuality

Slide 20

Supports

- Avoid judgment and projection of personal values or discomfort
- Ensure the privacy of each child and adolescent
- Promote self-care and social independence among persons with disabilities
- Advocate for appropriate sexuality education
- Help provide knowledge and/or identify a source of information
- Lack of attention to issues of sexuality can lead to misinformation and problem behavior

Slide 21

Sex Education

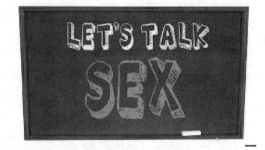

Slide 22

Childhood and Adolescence

Sex Education

- Provided by someone with special expertise
- Children with disabilities have the right to the same education about sexuality as their peers
- May need modifications
  - Simplifying information
  - Using special teaching materials as needed
    - Anatomically correct dolls
    - Role playing
    - Frequently reviewing and reinforcing the material
    - IEPs/IHPs should include provision of sexuality education

Slide 23

Childhood and Adolescence

Sex Education

- **Remember this is developmental and questions are completely normal**
  - Sexual thoughts or actions are not negative risk behaviors
- Parents/youth workers can help adolescents make safe and healthy choices regarding sexual behavior by:
  - Maintaining open lines of communication
  - Ensure access to appropriate information and resources
  - Adolescents with IDD need complete and accurate sex education so they can make informed decisions
- A team process
  - Planned and coordinated by support team
  - Parent input
  - Not just DSP

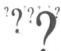

Slide 24

Childhood and Adolescence

Privacy

- Teach which behaviors are acceptable only do when they are alone
  - Provide guidelines about when
  - Review expectations
  - Guidelines about where
  - Ensure the guidelines are followed
- Identify and recognize cues in the environment (a closed door)
- Social cues for public settings
- Create cues for alone time (a sign on the door)

Slide 25

Childhood and Adolescence
Working Together

Empower young people to set limits
Assist lower-functioning individuals with achieving & maintaining privacy
When supervising or assisting with personal care:
- Be considerate
- Ask permission
- Remember they still need privacy
- Seek to minimize discomfort

Slide 26

Childhood And Adolescence
Gender Identity Issues

- In addition to physical development of sexual characteristics, exploration of sexual orientation
  - Refers to who one is emotionally and physically attracted
    - Heterosexuality
    - Homosexuality
    - Bisexuality

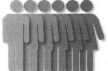

Slide 27

Childhood And Adolescence
Gender Identity Issues

Another important task is developing and maintaining intimate relationships

- Physical
- Emotional

Slide 28

Peer Pressure
Childhood and Adolescence

- Peer pressure is one thing that all teens have in common.
  - Need for acceptance, approval, and belonging is vital during the teen years.
  - Teens who feel isolated or rejected are more likely to engage in risky behaviors to fit in with a group
- During adolescence, begin to spend a lot more time with their friends, and less time with their family
  - More susceptible to the influences of their peers

Slide 29

Peer Pressure (continued)
Childhood and Adolescence

- Pressure isn't always negative
  - Pressure into negative behaviors
  - Away from positive behaviors
  - Positive influences, such as doing well in school, having respect for others and avoiding taking negative risks
- Handling peer pressure depends largely on how adolescents feel about themselves

Slide 30

Bullying
Childhood and Adolescence

- Childhood bullies are more likely to become young adult criminals than are non-bullies. Bullied children may grow up with diminished self-confidence
- Physical aggression: hitting, kicking, pushing, choking, punching
- Verbal aggression: threatening, taunting, teasing, starting rumors, fostering fear, hate speech.
- Exclusion from activities

Slide 31

Childhood and Adolescence

Bullying

- Done by someone with more power or social support to someone with less power or social support
- Often includes the abuser blaming the target for the abuse
- Often leads to the target blaming him or herself for the abuse.
- In most bullying situations, the target cannot stop the bullying by his or her own actions.

Slide 32

Exercise

- How do you think the way bullying is portrayed in popular tv shows/movies can affect a young person with IDD?

- What happened and how did the bullying resolve?

Slide 33

Childhood and Adolescence

Stop Bullying: What Doesn't Work

1. **Denial:** ("She would never do that;" "I'm sure he didn't mean to hurt you;" "Boys are just like that;" "Sticks and stones may break bones, but words will never harm")

2. **Telling the victim to solve the problem:** ("Just make sure you're never alone with that kid;" " Say no;" "Stand up for yourself and hit back ;" "Wear less revealing clothes;" "Pretend it doesn't bother you")

3. **Broad-brush educational efforts alone:** ("Soft is the heart of a child;" Sensitivity training; "Hands are for helping, not hurting")

Slide 34

Childhood and Adolescence

Stop Bullying – What Works

- **Consistent enforcement** of effective consequences which are **predictable, inevitable, immediate, and escalating**.
- **Monitoring** to make sure that consequences and education are effective.
- Effective **counseling** for youth who bully after enforcement of consequences has generated some anxiety.

Slide 35

Childhood and Adolescence

Stop Bullying – What Works
(continued)

- Effective support for targets, including **protection** from repeat victimization.
- **Empowering** bystanders to tell adults, support targets, and **discourage unacceptable behavior**.

Slide 36

Childhood and Adolescence

Gangs

- Gang violence has spread to communities throughout the world. In the US, these are the statistics:
  - More than 24,500 different youth gangs around the country,
  - More than 772,500 teens and young adult members
- Teens join gangs for a variety of reasons.
  - Seeking excitement
  - Looking for prestige
  - Protection
  - Make money
  - A sense of belonging
- Few teens are forced to join gangs; most can refuse to join without fear of retaliation

Slide 37

Steps to Conflict Resolution

- **Set the stage.** Agree to try to work together to find a solution peacefully, and establish ground rules (e.g., no name-calling, yelling, or interrupting).
- **Gather perspectives.** Each person describes his/her perspective. Listeners pay attention to what the others say they want, and why.
- **Find common interests.** Establish points everyone agrees on. Identify common interests, can be as simple as a shared need to save face.
- **Create options.** Brainstorm possible solutions: both people gain something, think win-win!
- **Evaluate options.** Each teen discusses feelings about solutions. Negotiate to reach a conclusion acceptable to both.
- **Create an agreement.** The teens explicitly state their agreement and may even want to write it down.

Slide 38

Adolescent disorders

- Teens deal with related issues all the time; when it gets out of hand, then it's a disorder
- May manifest differently than with adults
- Common problems:
  - Eating disorders
  - Depression
  - Substance Abuse

Slide 39

Eating Disorders

- **Anorexia nervosa:**

Intense fear of becoming obese, does not diminish as weight is lost

Disturbed body image – claims to 'feel fat' even when emaciated

Loss of at least 25 percent of original body weight

Refusal to maintain normal body weight

- **Bulimia –**

Recurrent episodes of binge-eating (rapidly consuming large amounts of food in a short time)

often followed by purging – vomiting or laxatives

Slide 40

Childhood and Adolescence

Eating Disorders: Causes and Solutions

- Causes
  - Adolescent focus on body image
  - Cultural emphasis on appearances
  - Other unmet emotional needs
- Response
  - Requires formal treatment
  - May include: lectures, group therapy, assertiveness training, drug therapy, and nutritional counseling
- Cautions
  - Avoid arguing, you're not going to talk them out of it
  - Be careful to avoid criticism

Slide 41

Childhood and Adolescence

Early Onset of Mental Illness

- Environmental stress does not cause mental illness, but can trigger onset.
- Biological events, chemical imbalance or disturbance requires psychiatric treatment.
- Untreatable mental illness places children at the risk of developing severe forms as adults, more reluctant to seek proper treatment.
- Poor functioning in school, development, social relationships, family life.
- Therapy can support, but is insufficient to treat, many severe illness driven symptoms and behaviors.
- Observation is key to Dx: intensity, frequency, impact.

Slide 42

Childhood and Adolescence

Triggers for Emotional Crises

- Onset of illness (medical or mental)
- Birth of sibling
- Onset of puberty/adolescence
- Start or end of school
- Out of home placement
- Sex and dating issues
- Changes in staff & teacher relationships
- Surpassed by younger siblings or peers
- Inappropriate expectations of others
- Physical, sexual, or emotional abuse
- Illness/aging of parents
- Death of parent, caretaker, family member
- Loss of peer or roommate

Slide 43

Exercise

Consider wellness strategies you can use to support a young person with IDD who might experience one of the emotional crises listed on the previous slide. Discuss with the group.

Slide 44

Childhood and Adolescence

Child Adolescent Depression

- Not just bad moods and occasional sadness
- Serious problem that impacts every aspect of a teen's life
- Requires treatment, can lead to:
  - Problems at home and school
  - Drug abuse
  - Poor adjustment and self-image
  - Negative identity
  - Homicide, violence, or suicide

Slide 45

Childhood and Adolescence

Depression Signs and Symptoms

- Sadness or hopelessness
- Irritability, anger, or hostility
- Tearfulness or frequent crying
- Withdrawal from friends and family
- Loss of interest in activities
- Changes in eating and sleeping habits
- Restlessness and agitation
- Feelings of worthlessness and guilt

Slide 46

Childhood and Adolescence

Depression Signs and Symptoms
(Continued)

- Lack of enthusiasm and motivation
- Fatigue or lack of energy
- Difficulty concentrating
- Thoughts of death or suicide
- Physical complaints (far more likely in youth than adults)

Slide 47

Childhood and Adolescence

Warning Signs, Teen Suicide

- Talking or joking about committing suicide.
- Saying things like, "I'd be better off dead," or "I wish I could disappear forever."
- Speaking positively about death or romanticizing dying ("If I died, people might love me more").
- Writing stories and poems about death or dying.

Slide 48

Childhood and Adolescence

Warning Signs, Teen Suicide
(Continued)

- Engaging in reckless behavior or having a lot of accidents resulting in injury.
- Giving away prized possessions.
- Saying goodbye to friends and family in dramatic ways.
- Seeking out weapons, pills, or other ways to kill themselves.

Slide 49

Childhood and Adolescence
Talking Tips for Depressed Teens

- **Offer support**
  - Let them know you're there for them. Avoid asking lots of questions (teens don't like to feel patronized)
  - Make it clear that you're ready and willing to provide whatever support they need
- **Be gentle but persistent**
  - Don't give up if they shut you out
  - Talking about depression can be very tough for teens
  - Be respectful, show you are concerned and willing to listen

Slide 50

Childhood and Adolescence
Talking Tips for Depressed Teens
(Continued)

- **Listen without lecturing**
  - Resist criticizing or passing judgment; when they talk at least they are communicating
  - Avoid offering unsolicited advice
- **Validate feelings**
  - Don't try to talk them out of depression
  - Acknowledge the pain and sadness they are feeling
  - Make them feel like you take their emotions seriously

Slide 51

Childhood and Adolescence
Substance Abuse

- **Experimenting**
  - Teens may try alcohol, cigarettes, inhalants, or other drugs one or more times, but not go any further
  - Usually do not have any problems as a result of substance use
- **Substance abuse**
  - Experimenting leads to regular or frequent use
  - Substance abuse results in problems at home (more arguments), at school (such as failing grades), or with the law
- **Substance dependence (addiction)**
  - Physical and/or psychological dependence
  - Use takes up a significant portion of the teen's activities,
  - Continues despite causing harm, and is difficult to stop.
  - An ongoing, and possibly fatal, disease.

Slide 52

Childhood and Adolescence
Health Care

- Adolescents – facilitate a transition to more active role in healthy behavior, medication management, appointments
- Help young people to understand their disability or diagnosis and health concerns
- Identify reliable resources for further information
- Teach healthy lifestyle skills, promote wellness
- Empower them to be more involved in asking questions and making decisions
- Provide guidance in knowing how and when to acquire or decline further help and support

Slide 53

Childhood and Adolescence
Community Safety

- Who/What is dangerous?
    - Help identify potential danger & make decisions beforehand about safety and trust
    - Build awareness by reviewing everyday dangers often: fire safety, traffic, crime, internet threats, risk-taking behavior
    - Build confidence to act safely "in the moment"
        - Discuss potentially threatening situations
        - Practice or role play appropriate response
        - Review who/how to ask for help

Slide 54

Childhood and Adolescence
Safety Tips

- Teach the person to always let someone know where he/she is going and for how long
- Routines
    - Many children with IDD depend on routines
    - Avoid routines that others can predict to victimize the kids
- Talk about safety often

Slide 55

Potential Victimization

- Appearance of safety doesn't mean there is no threat

- Grooming– *the establishment of trust through repeated interaction to increase access to a potential victim and decrease likelihood of discovery.*

- Awareness
  - Can children recognize they are being "set-up"?
  - Are parents/care providers able to tell when children don't see it?
  - What "Don't Talk to strangers" means

Slide 56

Internet Safety

- Keep the computer in a high-traffic area
- Establish limits for which online sites children may visit and for how long.
- Remember that Internet technology can be mobile, so make sure to monitor cell phones, gaming devices, and laptops.
- Surf the Internet with your children and let them show you what they like to do online.
- Ask questions about their interests and have them show you what they are searching.
- Bookmark/shortcuts to apps and safe websites for immediate access.
- Continually dialogue with children about online safety.

Slide 57

Technology Safety

- Know who young people are communicating with online.
- Note numbers of outgoing/ingoing calls with no contact information.
- Open a family/group/house e-mail account to share with younger children.
- Brainstorm screen names and e-mail addresses that do not contain information about gender, identity, or location, and avoid being suggestive.

Slide 58

Childhood and Adolescence

More Technology Safety

- Teach children never to open e-mails from unknown senders and to use settings to block messages from people they do not know.
- Be aware of other ways children may be going online—with cell phones, laptops, or from friends' homes or the library.
- Remind children that anything they send from their phones can be easily forwarded and shared.
- Familiarize yourself with popular acronyms at sites like www.netlingo.com and www.noslang.com/.

Slide 59

Childhood and Adolescence

Social Networking: Benefits

Gain social confidence: more secure in new situations, such as going to college, joining a sports team, and meeting new friends.

Learn about his or her diagnosis and health needs.

Find support in online communities – especially true for kids who have unique interests or feel isolated.

Make friends who are interested in the same thing or may be dealing with similar issues.

Slide 60

Childhood and Adolescence

Social Networking: More Benefits

Keeping in touch with family members that live far away by sharing updates, photos, videos, and messages.

Be Creative sharing ideas or poetry, blogging or journaling.

Increasing media literacy and expand vocabulary and communication skills.

Generates topics for discussion in "live" conversations and with peers in school and other offline settings.

Slide 61

Supporting Young People to Develop Goals

Set realistic expectations – consider:
- Strengths, abilities, and interests
- Opportunities, resources, and feasibility

Be careful not to devalue someone's ambitions

Break larger goals into mini-goals or objectives
- See progress quickly
- Even on a daily basis if needed.

Establish incentives that are meaningful to the person

Be flexible: use setbacks as building blocks to modify goals or create new dreams (turn disappointment into opportunity)

MODULE VIII

Post-Test

Module VIII: Childhood and Adolescence

___ 1. Which of the following diagnostic sign is NOT a potential sign of a developmental delay in a newborn infant according to the American Academy of Pediatrics?
(a) Reaching for an object
(b) Lack of response to loud sounds
(c) No smile response
(d) Feeding difficulties

___ 2. Which of the following is a purpose of having recognized developmental milestones?
(a) To set instructional expectations for children
(b) They are a widely used diagnostic tool
(c) To give a general idea of the changes to expect as a child gets older
(d) They have no purpose

___ 3. What is the typical age of a toddler?
(a) 0 – 1 year
(b) 1 – 3 years
(c) 2 – 5 years
(d) 2 – 7 years

___ 4. Typical children learn how to manage wanting everything immediately. The developmental activity associated with this is:
(a) Attachment to Caregivers
(b) Developing sense of identity
(c) Developing empathy
(d) Delaying gratification

___ 5. Why is sexuality education important for youth with IDD?
(a) All sexual thought is inherently risky
(b) Youth with IDD are sexual beings
(c) They must be protected from all sexual activity
(d) It is not important

___ 6. Children with IDD are:
(a) More likely to be bullied than typical youth
(b) Never bullied because they are always monitored by adults
(c) Rarely bullied because society doesn't accept it
(d) Easily taught to stop bullying by teaching martial arts

___ 7. Which of the following is NOT a step in conflict resolution?
   (a) Gathering perspectives
   (b) Threatening violence
   (c) Gathering options
   (d) Creating an agreement

___ 8. Which of the following is a type of healthy risk taking?
   (a) Drug use
   (b) Self-mutilation
   (c) Smoking
   (d) None are

___ 9. Difficulties with self-esteem may include?
   (a) Body image
   (b) Shyness
   (c) Embarrassment
   (d) All of the above

___ 10. Which of the following is a central question in the development of identity?
   (a) Who am I?
   (b) What am I to do in life?
   (c) Both of these questions
   (d) Neither of those questions

Aging

Module IX

Pre-Test

Module IX: Aging

___ 1. Due to factors associated with their disabilities, as they age, people with IDD
   (a) Generally have greater need for support and experience greater health-related functional decline than do older people without IDD.
   (b) Generally have decreased numbers of medical problems than the general population.
   (c) Generally experience similar rates of psychiatric problems than the general population.
   (d) Are never able to learn new material.

___ 2. The World Health Organization acknowledges that for people with IDD
   (a) Old age begins at around age 50.
   (b) There is no generally accepted age which defines exactly when people become old.
   (c) Aging is a lifelong process of change.
   (d) b. and c. are correct.

___ 3. Aging, in any population, increases vulnerability to certain health issues. In people with IDD, vulnerability can be increased by
   (a) Genetic factors.
   (b) Institutional living.
   (c) Lack of education about health promotion and prevention.
   (d) All of the above.

___ 4. Age related issues more frequent in people with particular genetically based syndromes can include
   (a) Plantar fasciitis.
   (b) Hypermelatonia
   (c) Musculoskeletal disorders.
   (d) All of the above.

___ 5. As they age, the rate of psychiatric disorders for people who have IDD is
   (a) 2 to 4 times the rate of the general population.
   (b) The same as that of the general population.
   (c) Half that of the general population.
   (d) None of the above.

___ 6. Identify which of the following statements is false. Diagnosing dementia in a person with IDD can be complicated by
   (a) Difficulty the person may experience when answering questions about memory or higher cognitive functioning
   (b) Lack of reliable, standardized diagnostic procedures for dementia.
   (c) Mutations in genes that are related to brain activity.
   (d) Difficulty in establishing baseline for cognitive functioning and daily living tasks.

___ 7. What are key responsibilities for primary care and specialist health services?
   (a) Maintenance of the physical and mental health of people with IDD
   (b) Early detection and treatment of both physical and mental health problems
   (c) Both A and B
   (d) Neither A nor B

___ 8. Which of the following is NOT a possible social aspect of aging?
   (a) Loss of family and friends
   (b) Mental Status Examinations
   (c) Financial and estate management
   (d) Changing interests

___ 9. Which of the following is not a potential component for wellness?
   (a) Optimizing physical health
   (b) Managing chronic conditions
   (c) Promoting health
   (d) None of the above – all are potential components for wellness

___ 10. Which genetically based syndrome has not been proven to cause age-related health problems?
   (a) Down syndrome
   (b) Fragile X syndrome
   (c) Irritable Bowel syndrome
   (d) Cri-du-Chat syndrome

Slide 1

Module IX

Aging

Slide 2

Mental Wellness and Aging in People with Intellectual/Developmental Disabilities

Slide 3

The purpose of this module is to discuss mental wellness among persons with IDD who are aging, considering the experiences of typical persons as well.

Slide 4

Learning Objectives

- Define and describe the components of wellness as it relates to aging
- List the types of changes that occur for people as they age
- Explain the factors affecting people with IDD as they age
- Explain how to enhance supports in consideration of these factors and the IDD
- Describe the age-related health problems attributed to genetically based syndromes
- Describe dementia, the prevalence among people with IDD and the challenges in diagnosing
- Describe the psycho-social aspects of aging with IDD and how to support a person to maintain healthy psycho-social contacts

Slide 5

Aging

The WHO (World Health Organization) acknowledges that aging is a lifelong process of change and there is no generally accepted age which defines exactly when people become old.

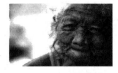

Slide 6

Aging

Understanding Aging

For some people, the types of changes that occur toward the end of their lives may require more care and support.

As people who have a dual diagnosis age, **understanding and supporting their mental wellness is crucial.**

Slide 7

A New Perspective — Aging

Clinical definition – "aging is a continuation of the developmental process and is influenced by genetic and other biological factors as well as personal and social circumstances."

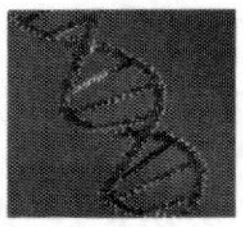

Slide 8

A Diverse Process — Aging

The accumulation of changes over time occur at different rates depending on an individual's genetics, environment, and lifestyle.

Physical and physiological changes make the body more susceptible to illness but no certain pathology is predictable without consideration to lifestyle variables. (Saxon et al., 2009)

Slide 9

Exercise

What words come to your mind when you hear the word "aging?"

Slide 10

Aging

Aging and IDD

Due to factors associated with their disabilities, people with IDD generally have poorer health, greater need for support, and experience greater health-related functional decline than do older people without IDD.

Slide 11

Aging

For some people who have IDD, aging can be complicated by the occurrence of what appears to be premature aging and shortened life expectancy; particularly for people with profound and multiple disabilities and frequently those with Down syndrome.

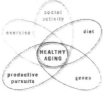

Slide 12

Aging

Aging in the General Population

Aging in the general population increases vulnerability to certain health issues:
- Memory and Alzheimer's disease
- Sensory problems: Eye and ear conditions
- Digestive and metabolic disorders
- Urogenital conditions such as incontinence and prostate cancer
- Dental conditions such as periodontitis, gingivitis and tooth loss
- Skin conditions – skin cancers, shingles, dry skin, pruritus, geriatric eczema

Slide 13

Concepts in Physical Aging

Skeletal system

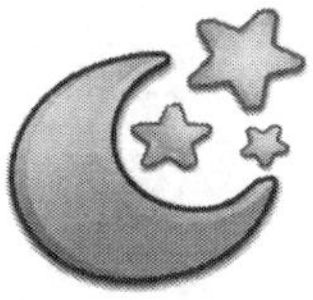

Nervous system

Physical abilities are compromised

Slide 14

Learning and Memory

Common myths and stereotypes have long implied that older adults are not able to learn new material or that poor memory is part of aging. (Saxon et al., 2009)

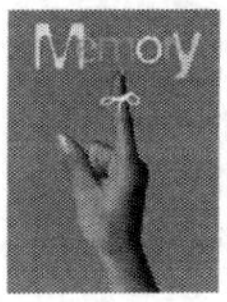

People continue to have different learning styles as they age.

Slide 15

Life Expectancy

As a result of advances in health care and community supports, life expectancy is increasing for people who have intellectual/developmental disabilities.

For example, life expectancy for people with Down syndrome has increased dramatically in recent decades - from 25 in 1983 to 60 today.

Slide 16

The Differences in Aging with an IDD

Aging

- Genetics
- Environmental Factors and Lifestyle
- Access to specialized health and mental health services for people who have IDD or dual diagnosis
- Communication
- Accelerated aging

Slide 17

Aging

Accelerated Physical Aging

There is evidence that people with IDD develop secondary conditions and diseases. As a result, they may age at a different rate than the general population.

Features of aging that can manifest as a gradual reduction in ability or capacity in an individual in the general population, can occur more rapidly in someone with IDD.

Slide 18

Aging

Other age-related health issues are more frequent in people with particular genetically based syndromes.

- Mitral valve prolapse and musculoskeletal disorders in people with Fragile X syndrome
- **Scoliosis in people with Prader-Willi syndrome**
- Recurrent upper respiratory and ear infections in people with Cri du Chat syndrome

Slide 19

Aging

For many intellectual/developmental disabilities with genetic etiology, there are known, existing predispositions for specified medical, mental health, and behavioral challenges.

Slide 20

Aging

The most commonly known of these is the increased risk of precocious aging, dementia, and increased sensory loss in people with Down syndrome.

Slide 21

Aging

The prevalence of certain mental health issues increases with aging, including anxiety, depression, dementia, and psychosis.

From the available research, it can be reasonably concluded that people who have IDD are more likely to develop a mental health issue as they age.

Slide 22

Prevalence of Mental Health Problems — Aging

The rate of psychiatric problems for people who have IDD is two to four times the rate of the general population as they age.

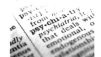

Slide 23

Dementia — Aging

The DSM 5 defines dementia as Neurocognitive Disorder. It involves the "loss of memory plus impairment in at least one other cognitive function, such as aphasia, apraxia, agnosia; and disturbance in executive function, which is severe enough to interfere with activities of daily living and represents a decline".

Slide 24

Dementia Prevalence Rate — Aging

22% of adults 40+ who have Down syndrome develop dementia.

The rate increases to 56% for adults 60+.

For individuals with other types of IDD the rate is comparable to that of the general population, 5% in adults 60+.

Slide 25

Challenges in Diagnosing Dementia

- Measuring decline in functioning
- Self-reporting observations
- No standardized criteria for dementia

Cooper, 1997

Slide 26

Case study: Maria is a woman with Down syndrome. She is in her 40s, and her health is failing. She suffers from digestive discomfort and sometimes has trouble hearing. She no longer has the energy to do the things she likes to do, and her favorite TV show, The Office, has gone off the air. Her life just seems to be slipping away. She gets crabby and takes her frustration out on staff, taking an occasional swing when she has energy and spitting at staff when she does not.

Exercise: Think about ways you could use these approaches to develop interventions to support Maria's wellness: Positive Behavior Supports, Mental health interventions, and Person Centered, Planning.

Slide 27

For people who have an intellectual/developmental disability, lifelong attention to preventable medical and mental health conditions is critical for healthy aging.

Slide 28

Best Practice Guidelines for Physicians — Aging

In 2011, Canadian Consensus Guidelines were developed for primary care physicians on evidence-based, best practice in preventative health care for people with IDD.

In 2014. these tools were adapted by Vanderbilt Kennedy University Center for Excellence in Developmental Disabilities for use within the US health care system.

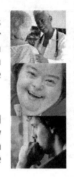

Slide 29

Primary Care Toolkit — Aging

The Canadian Primary Care Guidelines and Toolkit are available at:
http://www.surreyplace.on.ca/primary-care

The primary care tools adapted for use in the US health care system are available at:
http://vkc.mc.vanderbilt.edu/etoolkit/

Slide 30

The Social Aspects of Aging — Aging

As with all people, aging people with IDD deal with a variety of psychosocial changes and support as they age.

- increasing social isolation
- changing interests
- declining energy
- retirement

Continued.....

Slide 31

Continued...

- cognitive decline
- financial and estate management
- loss of family and friends
- grief management
- acceptance of mortality
- lack of meaningful work or hobbies

Slide 32

Social Value

Social value contributes to overall wellness for all people.

This includes people who have IDD who want to participate in and contribute to their communities in the same manner as all citizens.

Slide 33

Exercise

What social value did you experience from older people as you were growing up?
- Did you spend time around your grandparents?
- Were older people respected during your childhood?
- How can we ensure the people with IDD can continue to offer social value as they age?

Slide 34

Wellness — Aging

Wellness encompasses many components including:
- Promoting health and preventing illness, disease, and injury
- Optimizing mental and physical health
- Managing chronic conditions
- Engaging with life

Slide 35

Wellness — Aging

Key responsibilities for primary care and specialist health services:

1) Maintenance of the physical and mental health of people with IDD

and

2) Early detection and treatment of both physical and mental health problems

Slide 36

Working Together — Aging

As people who have IDD age, there is ongoing need for collaborative supports and services to address the needs of the person in this stage of life to ensure that wellness is assured as an accepted part of aging for this population.

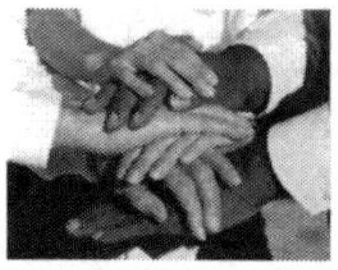

Post-Test

Module IX: Aging

___ 1. Due to factors associated with their disabilities, as they age, people with IDD
   (a) Generally have greater need for support and experience greater health-related functional decline than do older people without IDD.
   (b) Generally have decreased numbers of medical problems than the general population.
   (c) Generally experience similar rates of psychiatric problems than the general population.
   (d) Are never able to learn new material.

___ 2. The World Health Organization acknowledges that for people with IDD
   (a) Old age begins at around age 50.
   (b) There is no generally accepted age which defines exactly when people become old.
   (c) Aging is a lifelong process of change.
   (d) b. and c. are correct.

___ 3. Aging, in any population, increases vulnerability to certain health issues. In people with IDD, vulnerability can be increased by
   (a) Genetic factors.
   (b) Institutional living.
   (c) Lack of education about health promotion and prevention.
   (d) All of the above.

___ 4. Age related issues more frequent in people with particular genetically based syndromes can include
   (a) Plantar fasciitis.
   (b) Hypermelatonia
   (c) Musculoskeletal disorders.
   (d) All of the above.

___ 5. As they age, the rate of psychiatric disorders for people who have IDD is
   (a) 2 to 4 times the rate of the general population.
   (b) The same as that of the general population.
   (c) Half that of the general population.
   (d) None of the above.

___ 6. Identify which of the following statements is false. Diagnosing dementia in a person with IDD can be complicated by
   (a) Difficulty the person may experience when answering questions about memory or higher cognitive functioning
   (b) Lack of reliable, standardized diagnostic procedures for dementia.
   (c) Mutations in genes that are related to brain activity.
   (d) Difficulty in establishing baseline for cognitive functioning and daily living tasks.

___ 7. What are key responsibilities for primary care and specialist health services?
   (a) Maintenance of the physical and mental health of people with IDD
   (b) Early detection and treatment of both physical and mental health problems
   (c) Both A and B
   (d) Neither A nor B

___ 8. Which of the following is NOT a possible social aspect of aging?
   (a) Loss of family and friends
   (b) Mental Status Examinations
   (c) Financial and estate management
   (d) Changing interests

___ 9. Which of the following is not a potential component for wellness?
   (a) Optimizing physical health
   (b) Managing chronic conditions
   (c) Promoting health
   (d) None of the above – all are potential components for wellness

___ 10. Which genetically based syndrome has not been proven to cause age-related health problems?
   (a) Down syndrome
   (b) Fragile X syndrome
   (c) Irritable Bowel syndrome
   (d) Cri-du-Chat syndrome

Module X

Inter-Systems Collaboration

Pre-Test

Module X: Inter-Systems Collaboration

___ 1. People with a dual diagnosis generally _____.
   (a) Easily fit into the ID-DD system
   (b) Easily fit into the MH system
   (c) Can never fit into either system
   (d) Experience difficulty fitting into both systems

___ 2. Services for people with a dual diagnosis need to be _____.
   (a) Based primarily on the mental health concerns
   (b) Based primarily on the level of ID
   (c) Based primarily on a comprehensive assessment
   (d) Based primarily on what services are available

___ 3. Intersystem collaboration means: _____.
   (a) Interacting with your agency colleagues
   (b) Interacting with the person being served
   (c) Interacting with staff from other systems
   (d) Interacting with the individual and his or her family

___ 4. The purpose of a Dual Diagnosis Task Force includes _____.
   (a) Gathering relevant information to analyze strengths/weaknesses
   (b) Building an international headquarters for people with a dual diagnosis
   (c) Using the courts to catalyze change
   (d) Protecting persons with a disability abroad

___ 5. Lack of strategic planning has led to a "silo system" which _____.
   (a) Confines people with a dual diagnosis to small areas
   (b) Results in access barriers to required services
   (c) Ensures that people can escape the hustle and bustle of the city
   (d) Provides a plan to use state agencies as support

___ 6. The MH and IDD systems _____.
   (a) Always actively collaborate for betterment
   (b) Will collaborate if the person requires treatment
   (c) May work together if the person pursues
   (d) Often do not collaborate, fostering the divide between them

___ 7. Co-occurring disorders should be treated as _____
   (a) Multiple primary disorders with each requiring active treatment
   (b) By the severity of the disorder with the more severe being treated first
   (c) By the severity of the disorder with the more mild disorders being dealt with first
   (d) There is no such thing as co-existing disorders

___ 8. The goal of community collaboration is to _____.
   (a) Build a more effective system for individuals
   (b) Raise awareness for individuals within a community
   (c) Improve access to and availability of human services
   (d) All of the above.

___ 9. A holistic approach to care and treatment requires _____
   (a) A focus on a mental health approach
   (b) A focus primarily on developmental disabilities
   (c) Both a focus on mental health and developmental disabilities
   (d) Neither a mental health nor a developmental disabilities approach

___ 10. Systems that are important for people with disabilities _____
   (a) Are strictly limited to medical care
   (b) Mostly involve home and family life
   (c) Should not be limited to any one area
   (d) Should focus on housing and noting else

Slide 1

Module X

Inter-Systems Collaboration

Slide 2

Inter-Systems Collaboration

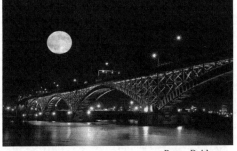

Peace Bridge,
Niagara Falls
USA/Canada

Slide 3

Learning Objectives

- Articulate how limited collaboration between mental health and IDD systems can result in barriers to service delivery.
- Recognize that assessment of individual need is at the center of effective person-centered service planning for individuals with MI/IDD.
- Explain how communication, cooperative relationships, and knowledge of service delivery are key to supporting someone with IDD/MI.
- Identify the 4 planning and practice elements essential to working together, and the factors that make each of these achievable.
- Describe the purpose, stakeholders, and potential roles of a Dual Diagnosis Committee.

Slide 4

Introduction

- Barriers to Service Delivery
- Principles in Service Planning
- Guidelines for Emergency Responders
- Community Collaboration and Teamwork
- A Framework to Promote Cross System Collaboration
- Service Planning Recommendations

Slide 5

Barriers to Service Delivery

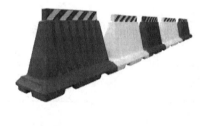

Slide 6

Dual Diagnosis Policy Barriers

The Typical Picture:

Individuals with MI and IDD are among the most challenging persons served by both MH and IDD Service Delivery Systems.

Slide 7

Dual Diagnosis Policy Barriers

The Typical Picture:

- Failure to plan services
- Failure to fund flexible services
- Failure to obtain technical assistance

Slide 8

Dual Diagnosis Policy Barriers

The Typical Picture:
- MH providers perceive that they do not have the skills to serve adults or children with a dual diagnosis.
- IDD providers do not understand the services that the MH sector offers.
- MH providers do not understand the services that the IDD sector offers.

Slide 9

Dual Diagnosis Policy Barriers

MH System	IDD System
Short term episodic treatment	Services/supports over lifetime
Focus on psychiatric needs	Emphasis on direct support
Recovery model	Self Determination
Local authority	State authority
Medication Treatment	Behavioral Support (PBS)
Consumer/Client/Patient	Self – Advocate/ Consumer

⟵ Little Collaboration ⟶

Slide 10

Principles & Practices in Intersystems Service Planning

Slide 11

Dual Diagnosis Planning Principles

- Co-occurring disorders should be treated as multiple primary disorders, in which each disorder receives specific and appropriate services.
- Collaboration of appropriate services and supports must occur as needs are identified.
- Services provided to the individual are consistent with what the person wants and what supports are needed.

Slide 12

Dual Diagnosis Planning Principles

- Services are determined on the basis of comprehensive assessment of the *needs* of each individual.
- Services are based on individual needs and not solely on either MH or IDD diagnosis.
- Emphasize early identification and intervention.

Slide 13

Dual Diagnosis Planning Principles

- Involve the person and family as full partners.

- Coordinate at the system and service delivery level.

Slide 14

Dual Diagnosis Planning Principles

The system recognizes and values the long-term cost effectiveness of providing best practice services and supports for persons with co-occurring disorders.

Slide 15

Community Collaboration and Teamwork

Knowledge of Service Systems

People with IDD and mental health needs are often served by different programs. Treatment and care is enhanced when knowledge and efforts across systems are considered in a community-based approach. This includes:

- knowledge about state and provincial systems and services including education, health care, DD/IDD services, mental health services, inpatient referral process, the justice system, foster care, youth services, community disability services, transportation and employment
- knowledge on issues and practice related to informed consent to protect an individual's confidentiality to promote both privacy and respect for the client

Slide 16

Community Collaboration and Teamwork

Communication with Multiple Systems

Supporting someone with IDD/MI

- Communicate signs and symptoms of individuals' mental health concerns to others across multiple systems.
- Articulate knowledge about the treatment history and current support needs of individuals
- Can present a professional approach to working with others across systems for the benefit of individuals, including sensitivity to the policies and procedures of other professionals
- Can convey complicated information sensitively to others who need to know about an individual's needs and supports, particularly during a behavioral or medical crisis

0Slide 17

Community Collaboration and Teamwork

Facilitating Positive and Cooperative Relationships

- Demonstrates ability to navigate recommendations between systems (e.g., psychiatrists and other health professionals, employment, residential settings)
- Demonstrates the ability to build positive and cooperative relationships with other health and mental heath professionals
- Can work positively with multiple systems as a collaborative and cooperative member of the team
- Maintains professional and empathetic communication and partnership with family members and friends of individual
- Recognizes family members as integral partners in support and gathers input from them
- Demonstrates problem solving and teamwork skills

Slide 18

Working Together

Effective Planning and Practice Elements

1. Leadership
2. Effective Staff
3. Effective Treatment
4. Staff Training

Slide 19

Effective Planning and Practice Elements

Working Together

1. Leadership
   - Commitment
   - Clear lines of authority
   - Commitment to collaboration
   - Focus on the Individual

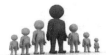

Slide 20

Effective Planning and Practice Elements

Working Together

2. Effective Staff
   - The right person
   - The right match
   - Build trust, dependability
   - Focus on the Interystem
   - Collaboration System
   - IDD/MH interface

Slide 21

Effective Planning and Practice Elements

Working Together

3. Effective Treatment
   - Appropriate psychiatric diagnosis
   - Effective medication treatment if needed
   - Positive behavioral supports
   - Effective treatment strategies such as DBT, CBT

Slide 22

Working Together

Effective Planning and Practice Elements
4. Staff Training
- DSP
- Clinicians
- Service Coordinators

Slide 23

Inter-Systems Collaboration

Purpose/Function of A Dual Diagnosis Committee
- Gather relevant data/information
- Identify strengths in service delivery systems
- Identify challenges/gaps in service delivery system
- Develop solutions to address challenges and gaps

Slide 24

Inter-Systems Collaboration

Stakeholders from other than MH & IDD systems could be included as appropriate. These include, but are not limited to, representatives from:

- Substance Abuse
- Justice
- Health Department
- Social Services
- Parents
- Consumers
- Advocacy Organizations
- Special Education
- Early Intervention
- Child Welfare
- Coordinated Children's Services
- Service Providers
- Senior Services

Slide 25

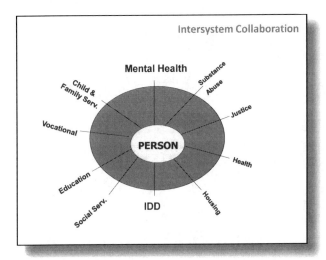

Slide 26

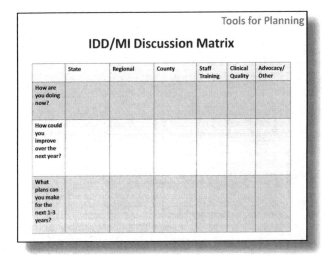

Slide 27

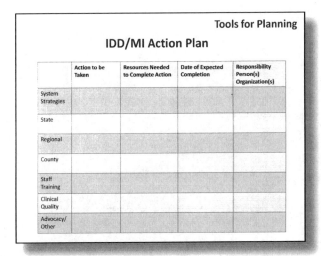

MODULE X

Post-Test

Module X: Inter-Systems Collaboration

___ 1. People with a dual diagnosis generally _____.
  (a) Easily fit into the ID-DD system
  (b) Easily fit into the MH system
  (c) Can never fit into either system
  (d) Experience difficulty fitting into both systems

___ 2. Services for people with a dual diagnosis need to be _____.
  (a) Based primarily on the mental health concerns
  (b) Based primarily on the level of ID
  (c) Based primarily on a comprehensive assessment
  (d) Based primarily on what services are available

___ 3. Intersystem collaboration means: _____.
  (a) Interacting with your agency colleagues
  (b) Interacting with the person being served
  (c) Interacting with staff from other systems
  (d) Interacting with the individual and his or her family

___ 4. The purpose of a Dual Diagnosis Task Force includes _____.
  (a) Gathering relevant information to analyze strengths/weaknesses
  (b) Building an international headquarters for people with a dual diagnosis
  (c) Using the courts to catalyze change
  (d) Protecting persons with a disability abroad

___ 5. Lack of strategic planning has led to a "silo system" which _____.
  (a) Confines people with a dual diagnosis to small areas
  (b) Results in access barriers to required services
  (c) Ensures that people can escape the hustle and bustle of the city
  (d) Provides a plan to use state agencies as support

___ 6. The MH and IDD systems _____.
  (a) Always actively collaborate for betterment
  (b) Will collaborate if the person requires treatment
  (c) May work together if the person pursues
  (d) Often do not collaborate, fostering the divide between them

___ 7. Co-occurring disorders should be treated as _____
   (a) Multiple primary disorders with each requiring active treatment
   (b) By the severity of the disorder with the more severe being treated first
   (c) By the severity of the disorder with the more mild disorders being dealt with first
   (d) There is no such thing as co-existing disorders

___ 8. The goal of community collaboration is to _____.
   (a) Build a more effective system for individuals
   (b) Raise awareness for individuals within a community
   (c) Improve access to and availability of human services
   (d) All of the above.

___ 9. A holistic approach to care and treatment requires _____
   (a) A focus on a mental health approach
   (b) A focus primarily on developmental disabilities
   (c) Both a focus on mental health and developmental disabilities
   (d) Neither a mental health nor a developmental disabilities approach

___ 10. Systems that are important for people with disabilities _____
   (a) Are strictly limited to medical care
   (b) Mostly involve home and family life
   (c) Should not be limited to any one area
   (d) Should focus on housing and noting else